PSYCHOLOGICAL PERSPECTIVE OF HIV AND AIDS

By the same Author

- Modern Psychological and Scaling Methods and Experimentation
- Statistical Methods in Psychological and Educational Research
- Contemporary Fields of Psychology and Experiments
- Experimental Psychology with Advanced Experiments (in Two Volumes)
- Modern General Psychology (Revised Edition)

About the Editor

M. Rajamanickam, formerly Professor and Chairman of the Department of Psychology and Dean, Faculty of Education, Annamalai University, is presently Founder-Director of the Institute of Community Guidance and Research. He was elected to the Syndicate of the Annamalai University for three times. Also, Dr. Rajamanickam has been the Founder-Editor of the Journal of Community Guidance and Research for 20 years. He has to his credit a good number of books, both in English and Tamil, on psychological themes.

PSYCHOLOGICAL PERSPECTIVE OF HIV & AIDS

Edited by
DR. M. RAJAMANICKAM, M.A., M.Litt., Ph.D.
Formerly Dean, Faculty of Education
and Professor and Head of the Department of
Psychology, Annamalai University

CONCEPT PUBLISHING COMPANY, NEW DELHI-110059

Cataloging in Publication Data—DK
Courtesy: D.K. Agencies (P) Ltd. <docinfo@dkagencies.com>

Psychological perspective of HIV & AIDS /
edited by M. Rajamanickam.
p. cm.
Contributed articles.
Includes bibliographical references (p.)
Includes index.
ISBN 8180692280

1. AIDS (Disease). 2. AIDS (Disease)—India. 3. HIV Infections. 4. HIV Infections—India. 5. AIDS (Disease)—Patients—India—Psychology. I. Rajamanickam, M. (Muniappa), 1925-

DDC 616.979 200 954 21

ISBN 81-8069-228-0

First Published 2006

Published and Printed by
Ashok Kumar Mittal
Concept Publishing Company
A/15-16, Commercial Block, Mohan Garden
New Delhi-110059 (India)

Phones: 25351460, 25351794
Fax: 091-(11)-25357103
Email : publishing@conceptpub.com

Preface

People in almost all the countries are threatened by an infectious disease called HIV-AIDS which has made its emergence around 1970s. The HIV-AIDS is created by man, and it is sexually transmitted disease caused by a virus named human immune deficiency virus. Researches are going on for the past twenty-five years to find out how it is caused and where it originated. There are few controversial views with regard to its cause and origin and development. Several views were expressed, but there is no unanimously accepted view about it. Experiments on this issue cannot be conducted just like all other diseases in the medical, chemical and biological fields. Because it is a very sensitive problem rooted in human sexual behaviour.

But how this human sexual behaviour has become so dangerous and fatal? Human sexual activity is not new in its function. It was going on right from the time when man was born in this world. There were sex diseases like the venereal disease, (VD); Syphilis and Gonorrhea. Millions of men died of these diseases and man was able to conquer these diseases by discovering suitable medicines and methods of treatment. This disease, the HIV-AIDS cannot be said as absolutely new in origin. It must have been from the advanced stage of the existing diseases like syphilis or venereal disease or something else, with the infection of some chemical substances like the anthrax. But it is for the medical, and biological and chemical scientists to trace out the correct origin of this disease.

The alarming consequences caused by the AIDS made the World Nations to awake and take quick precautionary measures to curb this disease from spreading out any further. The United Nations observers are visiting various countries to study the situation and provide funds for treatments and medicines. Enormous amount of publicities are made to make people to become aware of the dire consequences of the disease and to keep them away from the infectious disease.

AIDS control organizations started in many of the countries like China, Russia, African countries, India, Sri Lanka and in some of the South Eastern countries. India is one of the countries very much infected with AIDS. In India, Tamil Nadu tops the list. The other States most infected by this disease are Maharashtra, Andhra Pradesh, Karnataka and Manipur. Since it is becoming a very big social problem every person should come forward to contribute his might for the eradication of this disease and make India as the AIDS free nation.

Shri Ashok Kumar Mittal of Concept Publishing Company deserves all appreciations for having taken very much interest in bringing out this book at this juncture as the subject matter the HIV-AIDS is receiving paramount importance all over the world. Since the conditions prevailing in India are becoming the gravest challenges for the Medical, Chemical, Biological and Psychological Scientists in their intervention programme of preventing this most dangerous infectious disease, this book would certainly serve a very useful purpose among all sections of the people in our country.

M. Rajamanickam

Contents

1

A Psycho-Social Study of the AIDS and the Drug Abuses

M. RAJAMANICKAM*

INTRODUCTION

Life is full of inseparable illness and it exists in all species even in bacteria and at the molecular level. Illness is a subject matter coming within the scope of biology, medicine, biochemical, anatomy, psycho-biology, psychosomatic and psychopathology. Over centuries learned people who tried to study illness had no other means of doing so than to describe what they saw, recorded and what the patient said about his feelings, try to put together the symptoms to make a seemingly coherent whole, treat this collections of knowledge as an entity and give it a name. The study of symptoms had to be linked to visible and palpable effects on organs. One of the most remarkable examples is that of tuberculosis. During the first and second quarters of twentieth century it has played havoc. Other discrepancy which is more disturbing is disorders which did not reveal themselves anatomically. Disorders of human machine are caused in most cases by the virus, a bacterium or a parasite. These are the external agents that have entered the body by some means or other and cause troubles.

* Formerly Dean, Faculty of Education and Professor and Head of the Department of Psychology, Annamalai University.

Human race from time to time was put into untold miseries and mass death incidences due to highly infectious diseases. It is recorded in the history that diseases like plague, yellow fever, cholera, flu, tuberculosis, cancer all had their shares in killing people all over the world in the past. Just like new scientific inventions and discoveries, fatal diseases are also emerging at times. Tuberculosis is a bacterial infection that is diminishing today because of an intelligent policy of prevention is being pursued and anti-biotics are employed. It is known that virus diseases give more cause for concern.

Biological scientists ascertain that human longevity has been increased on the average all over the world during the course of 50 years, that is from 1900 to 1950. In European countries in 1900 the average age of death was 40 years and in 1950 it was 57 years. Thus during the course of 50 years 17 years of human longevity has been increased. This prolongation of life was no doubt attributed to the progress of medicine and hygienic way of life, food and clean habits. It is also observed that certain diseases were disappeared and some were made very rare and reduced the seriousness in the case of others. The other important reason could be the social progress and the psychological outlook which enabled people more and more to get the benefit from the application of scientific knowledge. All the statistics show that life today is much longer than it was in the past.

Man's desire to live longer and better resulted in inventing and discovering powerful medicines and methods of treatment. Noticeable results, no doubt were achieved at all levels. But on the other side, there are certain serious diseases appear time to time and make people perish in large numbers. Some of them were found to be very difficult to treat and save people from death. But, however, man was able to conquer some of them by inventing suitable medicines and methods of treatment and was able to control some of the deadliest diseases like yellow fever, tuberculosis and cancer.

EMERGENCE OF THE AIDS

The other dreadful and highly infectious disease that is spreading very fast all over the world after 1970s and threatening human race with dire consequences today is the AIDS. Unlike the tuberculosis and cancer it has puzzled and baffled the chemical and the medical scientists and they are hard trying to find out suitable medicine and methods of treatment for his. It is new disease created by men and women and the correct root cause of it is yet to be traced. Information about this disease was available only from 1980s. But it was somewhat traced in 1979 in America from the Ugandian blood sample drawn in 1972.

Experts say that it is a sexually transmitted disease (STD) and, therefore, it finds its origin in human sex. Research results on this available so far were not able to provide any accurate information as to how this disease finds its origin in human sexual activities. The reliable information available is that AIDS is caused by a virus called Human-Immune-deficiency Virus (HIV) and AIDS is an abridged form for Acquired-Immune-Deficiency Syndrome. Ho and his associates (1985) were the first to isolate and identify the HI virus from the cerebrospinal fluid and neural tissues. Ho's patients have demonstrated certain neurological symptoms. These symptoms were quite similar to the symptoms exhibited by Nurnberg's patients which had the characteristics of what is known as AIDS dementia complex (ADC). This was the first evidence to conclude and to show that the HI virus is capable of crossing the brain-blood barrier which is considered to be the defence mechanism. This defence mechanism normally permits only oxygen, nutrients and waste to pass through between the blood vessels and the cerebrospinal fluid. If the HI virus gets access directly to the brain to cause ADC it is very strange. The HI virus somehow is able to contact the brain and becomes responsible for the cause of the ADC.

The human body has certain capacity to resist anything that is disagreeable or harmful or any germ that may cause some disease. The body is protected from some disease by some kind of energy which we may technically call immunity. This immunity is a system in the body to protect it and this may become deficit. When this deficiency takes place in the body to a considerable extent certain symptoms begin to appear. The word syndrome refers to a group or pattern of symptoms which occur together in a disease and represent the typical picture of the disease. But in the case of AIDS the group of symptoms refer to a group of diseases which are stated as the AIDS related complex (ARC).

Since the HI virus is responsible for destroying the immunity system of the body and should have come from outside through some source, it is stated as 'Acquired'. Once the AIDS virus of HIV gets into the body it starts attacking the helper cell, lymphocyte (T-4) of the immune system and destroys it. This is how the AIDS virus of HIV begins to function and how a person gets contact with AIDS and when the immune system is fully destroyed he becomes the victim of the AIDS.

One source of information as given by Pushpa Khurana (1989) is that the AIDS was prevalent in Africa among the green monkeys long long ago. It might have been transferred to human beings in Africa in two possible ways. The African tribal people might have been eating the green monkey's flesh and might have contracted the AIDS from these green monkeys. Or the tribal people might have been bitten by these green monkeys and might have contracted the AIDS through blood. Later on when the Africans were migrated to America they carried the AIDS with them and when there was an intermixture of races it has spread out first among the Africans and later on to all other races in America.

The Human-Immuno-deficiency-Virus (HIV) is a highly infectious one, differs from bacteria in various ways. It is so minute that it even passes through the filter paper. The important characteristic of this virus is that it attacks the helper cell (T-4) and skilfully manages to get into the helper cell, lymphocyte, (T-4) slowly. Even though the helper cell (T-4) resists the virus with all its might and at last it gets exhausted and it dies ultimately and the virus gets into the blood and attacks other helper cells (T-4) and destroys them. This process of function of the virus HIV is continued till the helper cell's (T-4) immune system is fully destroyed. At this stage the person becomes fully infected with the virus and becomes a full fledged (AIDS) patient. The duration between the time the virus HIV enters the helper cell (T-4) and the time the person develops the AIDS varies from person to person depending upon the resistance the helper cells put up against the virus and it can be prolonged even up to 4 to 8 years. Therefore, the struggle between the helper cells and the HIV is a struggle between survival and death of the person who is exposed to the HI virus.

Nurnberg *et al.*, (1984) in their studies have observed that the AIDS attack the central nervous system which leads to sometimes loss of memory and lack of concentration. This takes place sufficiently prior to the appearance of the symptoms of the AIDS related illnesses. In one of the recent studies Navia and others (1986) found that on examining seven dead bodies of the AIDS patients there were less than ten per cent of the patients had normal brains and most of them had the AIDS Dementia Complex (ADC) which is a disease having disintegrating effect upon memory, thought process, judgement and motor coordination. Now it is believed that these are caused by the HI virus.

An individual under severe emotions, social and physical duress if diagnosed with the AIDS will exhibit symptoms of depression, generalized malaise and forgetfulness. Actually in the beginning the medical professionals have stated this state of affair as psychological. But later on it was viewed that it is an organic mental syndrome, one of the facets of HI virus. It was Nurnberg *et al.*, (1984) have first discovered that the AIDS patients had organic mental syndrome caused by the HI virus. In another study Ultmann and others (1985) have observed that the AIDS diagnosed children aged 2 years to 6 years have exhibited retardation in language and motor skills due to the development of the AIDS Demantia Complex (ADC). They state that even though death is not immediate for these people eventually they all die of this.

All those who have positive for HIV first develop a less severe AIDS related complex (ARC) which later on develop into AIDS within eight years. The AIDS' trouble aggravated because the people who are infected with the HI virus feel that they are healthy and not aware of their illness since they did not have the Elisa test to confirm their illness.

The root cause of other infectious diseases can be traced in the environmental pollution, food poisoning and germs. But the root cause of the AIDS from the information received so far through research findings seem to be in human sexual activities and through the drugs human beings consume and in the intravenous injections by unhygienic ways. It is also said that there is no medicine to cure the AIDS. Why were the scientists not able to find out suitable methods to treat this disease and to invent medicines in spite of spending millions of dollars and more than ten years of research on this?

1. The main reason for this has been that the disease AIDS was caused by human beings through abnormal sexual deviations and by drug dependence and drug abuses. Since the AIDS is a Sexually Transmitted Disease (STD) it is rooted in the promiscuous sex activities of heterosexual or homosexual in nature. There are greater chances to contract AIDS with greater number of sexual partners indiscriminately.

One of the important reasons the psychologists state for the infection of the dreaded disease, the AIDS is the attitudinal changes in different age groups toward premarital, permissive and promiscuous sexual relations. There are experimental evidences that the amount of education at the school and college level is positively associated with permissive attitudes toward premarital sex relations. Glenn and Weaver (1979) have observed in their nationwide study in United States that at each age level permissiveness increased as the educational level increased. The greatest change was found to be across the generations. The acceptance of premarital sex relations among the younger generation was found to be more than double as compared to the previous generations. Phillis and Gromko (1985) have observed in their study a most remarkable change in the behaviour of the males and females. The premarital sexual behaviour among the males and females was almost the same and the level was much more higher than the previous era. There was a marked increase in the incidence of premarital sexual activity among the West German students during the short period of 1966-1980. The study made by Clement *et al.*, (1984) confirmed similar studies made in the United States.

Studies of this type should be conducted in AIDS infected nations like India. From the evidences available Psychologists Davison and Neale (1990) conclude after making several studies that the generational change in attitudes and behaviour toward premarital and permissive sex relations and various kinds of promiscuous sexual activities – all contribute to the incidence of two sexually transmitted diseases. The first is genital herpes which involve painful blisters in the area of sexual contacts accompanied by itching, fever and headaches. The second is the more dreaded disease called the AIDS which stands as the great public health threat today.

Scholars who have studied this disease have stated that it is a very dreadful and frightening monster, fateful, painful, carries severe feeling of shame and guilt. They have also stated that there is no cure and no escape from this disease as there is no method and medicine to treat this. This kind of alarming picture of this disease brought out very big publicity for this disease and made people panic and it has also become the cause of the development of phobic neurosis. Anybody who is suspected of having AIDS is socially boycotted. A person who has been branded with the AIDS refuses to make his appearance in the public.

The AIDS does not cause death of the person immediately. But it has created a sense of fear in the minds of the people that it might cause sense of shame and social boycott which they consider worse than silent death. The physiological consequences may be painful feelings of severe type, but its psychological consequences are anxiety, depression, nervous tension, obsessive compulsive neurosis, sense of guilt and shame, resorting to excessive alcoholic habits and drug addiction, feelings of insecurity in life and phobic neurosis. Most of the patients exhibit all sorts of psychosomatic disorders.

Several studies in recent times have been conducted on AIDS. In one of the investigations it was observed that it involves the patient's race, colour, creed, eating and living habits, social life, sexual life and other contacts. The striking feature of the AIDS is that among the cases identified in 1979 most of them were homosexuals. Whether it is homosexual case or heterosexual, the virus transmission is taking place in the contact through semen or blood. The transmission is greater in the case of multiple sexual partners. Since sex is a function of feeling aspect and also very sensitive, if a person is aroused with strong sexual feeling nothing stands on the way except sexual activity.

Man's emotional reaction to sexuality is determined much more by psychosocial factors than biological needs. What one does, how often he does it, with whom and at what age? Changes in the people's sexual behaviour and their attitudes to various aspects of sexuality have been quite common. There has been shifts from time to time between restrictiveness and permissiveness and the reason for this has not been identified. Baron and Byrne (1988), who have studied this aspect very extensively state that in the present century radical changes have taken place in sex in the western civilization. This they termed as Revolutionary Changes in Sexuality or Sexual Revolution. The changes were toward greater sexual freedom, increased legal tolerance for sexual contents in books and magazines, motion pictures and television. This attitude was developed in the European Civilization after the World War I and gained strength steadily till the late 1970s. As a result of this Sexual Revolution, beginning with the first quarter of twentieth century, the European cultures have to embrace the sexually transmitted disease (STD) like the Genital Herpes and the AIDS in the last quarter of twentieth century. The death rate due to these diseases increased from 118 in 1981 to 16,000 in 1986 in United States. The alarming fact is that most of those dying of AIDS are young men and women in their most productive years. In the social realm, the fear of death seems to grip the people and the incidences of casual heterosexual and homosexual activities found to be declining. These incidences turned the tide of the European Sexual Revolution on the reverse and now the European cultures are witnessing a reverse movement to the sexual revolution and indications of backlash — a counter revolution to the sexual revolution. This is the beginning of changes in sexual attitudes. It is toward the restrictiveness from permissiveness in sexual relations.

2. The other possibility of transmission of HIV into the blood of other person is intravenous drug injection through the needle and syringe not properly sterilized and cleaned.

3. Further, the virus is also transmitted through the transfusion of infected blood. The infected blood transfusion may be given to any person who needed blood transfusion.

The person might be a man or woman or a child having good immunity in his or her body. But the blood bank had stored blood from a virus infected person without conducting proper test. Therefore, such people who had the infected blood transfusion, become victims of the HI virus and in the due course they develop the AIDS.

Apart from these three causes there are also other minor causes. They may be incidents involving bleeding cuts and wounds, bites, incidents involving saliva in kissing etc.

There are greater chances to assume that large number of AIDS cases might be through prostitutes. As they have sexual contacts with multiple partners, the prostitutes become the store house of HI virus. First, the AIDS was prevalent in America and Africa, but now it is spreading out to Burma, Thailand, Siam and India. In India, Maharashtra, Tamil Nadu and Manipur are notable AIDS infected areas.

AIDS AND TUBERCULOSIS

Studies on AIDS revealed also certain other informations related to the AIDS. Evidences were obtained that tuberculosis is spreading out rapidly along with HI virus which causes the AIDS. *The New Scientist* reported that in Zambia reactivated tuberculosis is found to be common among the people who had HI virus infection. In developing countries most of the people who live in congested areas were much infected by the tuberculosis germs. This is almost a matter of routine in life. It is very difficult to kill the dangerous intruder. The defence cells in the body cover themselves around them. But sometimes under certain conditions the TB germs break through the barriers, attack the body and make the person seriously suffer from the tuberculosis. In Tanzania where the HIV and tuberculosis are endemic, the tuberculosis cases are rapidly increasing. It is found that even in United States the infection of HIV causes more cases of tuberculosis. The infection of HIV and tuberculosis causes more death cases. In one of the studies made in Zaire it was observed that out of 198 patients who were suffering from HIV infection and tuberculosis 32 died within a year. Investigations reveal that those who were infected with HIV also were found to be suffering from tuberculosis.

AIDS AND CHILDREN

One may feel guilty to associate the AIDS with children. It may be also felt as sin to speak of it. The adult has every reason to justify for his/her contract the dreadful diseases. The adult might have contracted it consciously or due to certain unavoidable circumstances. The child has no such chances. But children die of AIDS. Children might have genetic deformities, like blindness, deafness, numbness, feeble mindedness and so on. To think of a child dying of infected with the deadly virus is something beyond imagination. *The Science Express* (1991) states that according to the observation made by the World Health Organization (WHO) AIDS is becoming the major cause of death of infants and children during 1990s and it is estimated that by the year 2000 ten million children will be infected with AIDS.

The WHO has reported that during the past ten years there were about 4 lakhs of cases of AIDS reported among the infants and children. They were all under five years of age. But most of these cases were from Africa. There were about seven lakhs of infants had been born all AIDS infected all over the world and most of them were from the developing countries by 1990. Michale Merson (1990), the Director of global programme on AIDS of WHO has stated in the United Nations-sponsored World Summit for children that "AIDS is a growing problem in children because it is a growing problem in women". He further states that if we could foresee the impact of the AIDS in 2000 governments will have to put AIDS prevention at the tip now. The WHO state that the key priority should be the preventive messages aimed at children building up strong health services in developing nations and to expedite the research works.

There is every possibility for the child to contract the AIDS virus from the mother. It may be through blood transfusion, and exchange of body fluids. Infection may also occur during pregnancy times, delivery times and also after birth of the child through breast feeding. Symptoms of AIDS in children may appear within six months of their birth. It was in the year 1983 that the presence of AIDS was first diagnosed in the United States. There were 321 cases of AIDS infected children under the age of 13 years. These children had the infection during pregnancy and 60 per cent of them died. The most important symptoms that appear in children who had the infection of the AIDS are, dry coughing, fever for long time and the reason for which not known, appearance of white spots in the mouth, indefinitely shaped mass of swelling in the neck, armpits or in the groin that will not disappear.

There may be certain surprising incidents in the development of the AIDS in children. Parents may be very healthy and free from any symptoms of the AIDS. But their children might have developed the AIDS. How is that? It is because that the parents on some occasion might have given blood transfusion to the child without proper testing of the blood. The blood bank might have stored infected blood which might have been the cause of the development of the AIDS in the child.

METHODS ADOPTED TO IDENTIFY THE AIDS

There are two important tests, namely Elisa test and the Western Blot Examinations which can identify the HI virus infected drug addicts. The Elisa test can ordinarily be applied without much expenses and the presence of an anti-body to Human-Immuno-Virus (HIV) in an individual can be detected. An anti-body is a process of resistance automatically generated in the body for fighting virus. If the resistance of the anti-body is strong then the virus might leave the body without causing the disease. The detection of the anti-body is the indication that the virus has entered in the physical system of the body. This is the limitation of the result of the Elisa test. Any further information on this, that is, whether the virus is still there can be had by conducting another test called the Western Blot Examination.

The Western Blot Examination is an advanced test which is intended to ascertain whether the HI virus is still present in the individual in whom the Elisa test was conducted. Thus, this test confirms the presence of the virus in the individual's body. But the presence of the virus does not mean that the individual is having the disease of AIDS. It may take three to four years for the disease to have full development. Sometimes it may also disappear without causing much serious conditions. But the Western Blot Examination is very costly and is not available at all medical centres.

AIDS AND DRUG ADDICTION IN INDIA

There are medical reports, often published, about the spread of the AIDS in India. The AIDS was first traced in Tamil Nadu in the year 1985. Medical test were started and continued since then. *The Science Notes* (1991) states that according to the Indian edition of the *British Medical Journal*, AIDS is slowly spreading in several parts of India. There were about 5,588 persons found to have the AIDS causing virus out of nearly 10 lakhs persons tested by the end of June 1991. The report states that there were at least 68 of them having the symptoms of the AIDS. In certain parts of India it was observed that there were drug addicts having the AIDS causing virus. The drug, opium was in usage among the saints in India for thousands of years. It was believed that man can go into transcendental meditation after consuming opium. But at present, opium is misused by evolving several derivatives from it. Now it is associated with the AIDS in India.

Asha Nehemiah (1991) reported that the myth that India is AIDS free is shattered and a staggering one million Indians are probably infected by the AIDS causing virus. The AIDS problem has been dismissed for some time stating that it is a disease confined to America and Africa. But it has infiltrated into the children, adolescents, adults and old people, virtually in every corner of this country. After eight to ten years from now, one million people who are already infected with HI virus will begin to display physical manifestations of AIDS, though now they appear to be healthy and unsymptomatic.

Jacob John (1991), a virologist, an ardent fighter of AIDS from Christian Medical College, Vellore has stated that no part of India is free of HIV infection. He said that it is known from the test that the hot spots of AIDS in India are Mumbai and its surrounding areas followed by Chennai and its surrounding areas. There are also HI virus infected cases in Delhi, Kolkata and Manipur and its surrounding areas.

One of the important causes of the AIDS mentioned above is the intravenous drug use. This practice is widely prevalent among the smokers and drug users. The smokers and drug users are not satisfied with their smoking of the drugs. They find that the ordinary way of smoking and the use of drugs do not give so much of kicking and also there is much wastage of the costly drug, the heroin. Therefore, they resort to the practice of intravenous injection of the drugs.

Heroin is a narcotic drug. The important characteristic of narcotic drug is that it relieves pain and induces sleep. The various narcotic drugs are the opium and its derivatives such as morphine, codeine, and heroin. Man has been using opium and its derivatives for more than 5000 years. Galen, a Greek physician who lived in second century A.D. considered that opium was the cure of all diseases. It is said that it resists poison and venomous bites, cures headache, deafness, epilepsy, loss of sight, loss of voice, asthma, coughs of all kinds, hard breathing, urinary complaints, fever and all epidemic diseases.

Opium derivatives are even used for some conditions. Galen had stated that opium is a mixture of 18 nitrogenic components and it is known as alkaloids. It is bitter in taste, very powerful sedative powder. It is also a pain reliever and named as morphine after the name of the Greek God of sleep, Morpheus.

Morphine is also converted into another powerful pain reliever called heroin. This was discovered by Heinrich Dreser. Boehm (1968) has stated that heroin was widely used in place of morphine for pain relief. Later on it was found to be very dangerous drug. Dreser, therefore, shortly after this discovered aspirin, an effective non-addictive pain reliever. At last heroin was removed from medical practice, but it is widely used by drug addicts.

Codeine is another alkaloid derived from opium as a pain reliever and it is also used in some cough syrups. Since these narcotic drugs are not available through legal sources they turn out to be illegal and brought under criminal acts.

Fort (1954) states that the narcotic drugs are used by the teenagers and young adults in most of the societies all over the world. Morphine and heroin are commonly used in smoking. It is by way of inhaling the bitter powder and sometimes by eating the addicts make use of them. These narcotics are also used by the way of injecting them directly into the large vein. Thus the use of narcotic drugs progressed from smoking to injecting into the bloodstream. The reason for taking heroin in this way is for its effects. It gives a sudden violent temporary feeling for few minutes and it is compared to the sexual organism—the greatest sexual pleasure in the enjoyment. This feeling may continue for 4 to 6 hours and the addict during this period is found to be very lethargic and even the bodily needs like food, water and sex are diminished and the person is in a state of pleasant feeling of relaxation, euphoria and reverie and also desires for the drug more and more as he cannot withdraw himself from that state. Withdrawing himself from that state is an agonizing experience for him. Therefore, the addict wants to have it again and again and thus he becomes a slave to the drugs.

There are also other drugs like barbiturates, cocaine and lysergic acid diethylamide-25 (LSD) which can induce hallucinations. But at present the most popular drug is the heroin which is widely used in Burma, Thailand and in some eastern parts of India. Heroin in India is sold to the addicts in Manipur, Mizoram and Nagaland, smuggled and brought from Sri Lanka and moved to other neighbouring states. In the first week of April 1991 about

38 kg. of Brown Sugar was captured by the Narcotic Control Bureau of Madras in a lorry sent from Bombay to Nagerkoil in Tamil Nadu. Drug smugglers use various methods to conceal the drugs. Heroin is moulded into different shapes and disguised in the form of decorative tiles, fish cakes etc.

Drug abuse or dependence may occur at any age. But it is most common during the periods of adolescence and young adulthood. The adolescents and young adults once if they experience the effect of the heroin or any other narcotic drug they become slaves to it. Amita Bhattacharya (1990) states that the drug addicts after some time, ultimately resort to regular intravenous injections of the heroin. Medical experts who went to Manipur from Kolkata to study the AIDS have observed in their tests that the AIDS causing virus was identified in the blood of a drug addict in the hilly province of Manipur. The area is close to eastern Burma. Then a series of Elisa tests and Western Blot Examinations were conducted by the Medical experts and the tests revealed that there were 805 persons who had become the victims of the HI virus. It will take some time for the virus to develop into fullfledged AIDS. Here the victims were the drug addicts who has 90 per cent pure heroin injected into their blood and most of the drug addicts in Manipur area were desirous of intravenous injection to smoking. The drug addicts in Manipur use the same syringes and needles among themselves for the intravenous injections of the heroin. This practice, even though unhygienic, helps them to avoid spending more money in purchasing packets of white sugar, supposed to be the costly heroin. Thus the practice of injecting heroin (white sugar) into their veins through the same uncleaned syringes and needles, shared by many addicts, contribute for rapidly spreading of the deadly virus (HIV). In Manipur area most of the drug addicts were those who became rich by illegal methods and they were between the age group of 15 and 35 years. The youngsters get money from their extremely affectionate parents who did nor know the consequences of their acts of benevolence. It was also observed that the main reasons for the youngsters (adolescents and young adults) for resorting to smuggling and involving themselves in transporting objectionable goods from place to place and making money out of it. These acts of the youngsters seem to be due to economic backwardness of the area, unemployment problems, insufficient industrial development and no means of keeping the unemployed youths engaged most of the times. These are also may be stated as some of the causes that are contributing indirectly to the development of AIDS.

According to the information available from Pal (1990) on drug addiction and AIDS there are about 15,000 drug addicts in Manipur areas and out of which about 7,500 are supposed to be the victims of AIDS. From these statistics it is clear that 50 per cent of the drug addicts were affected by the HI virus. The figures about the AIDS from Manipur areas as stated by the Kolkata Medical Experts are sufficient evidence to ascertain that the drug addicts have more chances to become the victims of HI virus. The drug addicts who resort to intravenous injections mix heroin (white sugar) in whatever water they find for their purpose. The water they use might contain all sorts of germs. If the drug addicts do not find water within their reach for their purpose, they never hesitate to use their urine as liquid and dissolve heroin in it and prepare the solution and get it injected.

The heroin addicts who are accustomed to these habits know well that they are sure to be the victims of the fatal disease. They also might know that they would be isolated and segregated from the society and put into shame and loss of self respect. But still they have no mind to give it up and get rid of the disease and death. Segregating the heroin addicts from the society and keeping them in isolation may have the advantage of preventing others from getting the chances of the infection of the HI virus. In Manipur area strange incidents are taking place. The drug addicts were questioned and assaulted by the villagers. The Epidemiological Team which visited certain areas in Manipur watched that a drug addict who was hiding in some place was stoned to death by the angry village people. This shows that the village people were aware of the consequences of drug addiction and the drug addicts are the carriers of the HI virus. Therefore, the village people in Manipur areas did not want to permit the drug addicts who were suspected of the HI virus infected to stay in their residential areas. Therefore, it is quite evident that there was tremendous amount of awareness among the village people in Manipur areas about the consequences of drug addiction and spread of the HI virus which causes AIDS. The Epidemiologists and the Virologists who have visited Manipur areas from Kolkata were able to conclude that about fifty per cent of the drug addicts might turn out to be infected with the HI virus. They were able to arrive at this conclusion only after conducting extensive tests on drug addicts. The source for such extensive test was that one of the blood samples received from Manipur Medical Centre was found to be a case of Human Immunodeficiency Virus (HIV) infection.

AIDS IN TAMIL NADU

Tamil Nadu is becoming more and more the AIDS breeding area, second to Maharashtra State. Everyday some news bits appear in Newspapers about the AIDS cases. Recently the *Express News Service* (1991) has reported that there were 27 HIV positives in 20 days. It is highly shocking to know that of the 27 cases 17 were blood donors, five of them had gone to sexually transmitted disease (STD) clinics and three of them had gone to TB clinics. These cases were detected from the people who went to hospitals for different ailments. The undetected HI virus infected cases may be many more.

In the same issue of the *Express News Service*, Sandhya Nammalwar (1991) under the title of 'AIDS threat looms large over Tamil Nadu' has written that the dreaded AIDS is fast catching up throughout the State and quite a number of people get affected by the HI virus. It has been estimated that in the middle of the year: 1991 there were about 1500 cases of HIV infected and by October 1991 the number of cases has increased to 2,308. But the number of positive HIV cases has gone upto 2500 in Maharashtra State. The Government of Tamil Nadu was not active on this so far, has suddenly become aware of the consequences of the dreaded disease and started drawing out strategies to deal with this problem. The Indian Council of Medical Research has supported the State Government for setting up the AIDS surveillance centre at the

Madras Medical College, Madurai Medical College, Institute of Child Health and at the Vellore Christian Medical College. Apart from these there are also zonal blood testing centre set up in eight places with Elisa testing facilities. But the Elisa testing centres at Stanley Medical College, Salem Government Hospital and Thanjavur Hospital are very rarely put to use. It seems that people in this State are still not aware of the AIDS and its consequences. Another possible reason for not making use of these facilities is that people who are infected with the HI virus have not revealed any symptoms of this disease as it will take some more time.

The World Bank Appraising Team has also visited to study the AIDS problem in Tamil Nadu. In addition to 65 million U.S. dollar aid to India for controlling the AIDS the World Health Organization (WHO) has also its budget plan for preventing and controlling the AIDS for 1991-92. Of the large number of people tested positive for HIV in Tamil Nadu, about 1060 are promiscuous heterosexual women, going to STD clinics, 822 are prostitutes in vigilance homes, about 350 are voluntary blood donors and paid donors and the rest of them are the relatives of the AIDS patients and TB patients. The HIV infected persons were first traced at Ulundurpet in Tamil Nadu when 10 of the 100 prostitutes were screened for AIDS in 1986. There were 14 full blown AIDS cases reported in Madras Government Hospital, six cases in Madurai and Vellore Hospitals.

Jacob John (1991) a well known virologist states that the areas like Vellore, Madurai and Salem are also HI virus infected areas. According to his statement it is known that the members of CMC's AIDS Team in North Arcot district have made the people to be aware of the deadlist diseases. The team made the medical community at Vellore, Ranipet, Ambur and Vaniambadi to be aware of this first. The other communities they have chosen are the college students, policemen, bus drivers and conductors and industrial workers and managers. The CMC's AIDS Team has also planned to introduce a new health education package in all schools in urban and rural areas.

It is learned that the Government of Tamil Nadu as a part of the Annual Plan of AIDS control has envisaged to set up of blood testing centres, conducting survey among the industrial workers, college students and lorry drivers and also contemplating on special health education programme for the risk groups ranged from 15 years to 50 years of age. It is important that the Government of Tamil Nadu should include the Policemen in the risk-group as the CMC's AIDS Team has done. The core groups for 12 districts which are being constituted seem to be having one STD specialist, one social worker and one health worker. The members of the core groups will be given training to explain the consequences of the HIV infection and the ways and methods of preventing and controlling the AIDS. But it is very unfortunate that the core groups lack the presence of psychologists who should be the important core group persons in dealing with the AIDS. The AIDS affected people will have no means of getting the disease cured by medical methods however advanced they are. But the AIDS can be prevented and controlled by psychological methods as it is a psycho-socio-physical problem.

PREVENTIVE MEASURES

From the foregoing discussions it is implied that it is very difficult to go for a cure of the AIDS. Medicines and methods of treatment of the AIDS are not in proper utility anywhere in the world. Now and then some research findings are published on AIDS, experiments are conducted on animals with some new medicines. Experiments on human beings to test the new AIDS vaccine which was developed by A European-based pharmaceutical firm yet to be conducted on a group of 30 volunteers, who are free from AIDS infection, at a low dosage level and after knowing the effect of the preliminary attempt, if found successful, then the other test at a higher dosage level on another 30 volunteers will be conducted. The vaccine will be administered on a large group of people if only the early tests were found to be activating the disease fighting system in the body of the volunteers. The pre-clinical test first was tried on two chimpanzees. But the effectiveness of the extensive test of the vaccine is still at hypothetical level.

It is known that researchers are now able to get details as to how the AIDS virus gets into the white cells of the human body. This has facilitated the scientists for the development of new drugs to prevent the virus that would cause AIDS. But the results of these recent researches are not likely to have any immediate effect upon the AIDS. The research findings published in the November 29th issue of the Journal, *Nature* (1990), according to Wayne Hendrickson of Columbia University, may provide only false hopes among the AIDS patients.

Scientists all over the world put up their efforts very seriously to control and prevent the AIDS. It is true that every research finding throws some new light on AIDS. But the AIDS virus makes its appearance in different forms causing also some other diseases. One of the recent discoveries is that a gene product called 'tat' of the AIDS virus (HIV) promotes the growth of tumour cells. It is quite similar to Kaposi's sarcoma—a malignant tumour in connective tissues. This is a kind of skin cancer resulted from the AIDS virus. In United States, it was found to be a rare disease associated with elderly men and it has been estimated that among the AIDS victims about 10 to 15 per cent of deaths were due to this skin cancer. This they were able to declare only after the emergence and the discovery of the AIDS virus. Therefore, it was found that there was direct link between the HI virus and cancer. On these contexts it is very difficult to conclude what type of medicine and treatment could be developed to deal with the AIDS virus. Prior to treat the AIDS with medicines and methods which are yet to come, it is better to deal it with easily available and possible methods.

It is always better and safe to keep ourselves free from infection of this deadliest disease rather than allowing ourselves to get infected and then going for the treatment and medicines. There are two important ways of approaching this serious problem as preventive measures. One is the psychological approach which is now practiced mostly in United States and in some of the European countries. The other one is the cultural approach which is specific to India.

The Psychological Approach

In tackling the AIDS there are two interrelated important characteristics which could be discussed psychologically. The first is that at present the AIDS is neither curable nor preventable by medical methods. Secondly, it is preventable only by psychological methods.

The main psychological approach to tackle the AIDS is to change the attitudes of the present generation of high-risk people towards the premarital, permissive and promiscuous sexual behaviour. Many of the present day biologists and medical scientists look at the AIDS purely as the consequences of biological needs. But there is something more deep in this. It is that man's desire to fulfil his biological needs is strongly influenced by the motives, beliefs and attitudes that he has developed at the given time in a given place. One of the most striking aspects of sexual behaviour is that it undergoes changes dramatically across the cultures and generations, Kelly (1986) states that some of the most powerful factors influencing sexual behaviour of human beings are not physiological but psychological. Human beings more respond to erotic fantasies than to hormone levels. Much of sexual behaviour of human beings is influenced by both external and internal sexual images in the forms of pictures and words. The external fantasies to which the human beings are exposed to are in books, magazines, movies and television. These external images become the cause of internal images and sexual thoughts and lead to sexual arousal and sexual dreams, (Byrne and Lamberth, 1971). The effects of erotic fantasies are always seeking for overt behaviour like sexual coercion, forcible sexual advance and rape.

The Indian scene in this context at present is on the reverse of what is happening in the United States and European countries. There is growing a strong tendency in the minds of the adolescents and youths in India for premarital and permissive sexual relations. The sexual revolution that took place in the European cultures in the first quarter of this century is facing a counter revolution now, in the fourth quarter. But, in India it is now emerging with all its vigour and valence. There are debates, discussion and symposiums on greater intermixture of boys and girls in the Indian soil. The youths, particularly the adolescent boys and girls make it as a right to fight for the unrestricted intermixture of sex and for sexual relations. Books and magazines with too much of sex oriented pictures and photographs attract the youth and the adolescents very much.

The vulgar sex themes of the Indian motion pictures and the television plays are guiding the present generation of youth and the adolescents towards the revolutionary changes in sexuality. The adolescent girls more than the boys become more revolutionary in getting rid of the parents' restrictiveness on them for free sexual movements. There are instances that the adolescent boys and girls taking the vulgar sex themes of the motion pictures and television plays as models, revolt against their parents and run away from homes and fall prey to evil temptations of various types. There are criticisms, appeared (1991) from the Doordarshan audience condemning the Madras Doordarshan for telecasting the Tamil movie, '*Aligal Oivathilai*'. One letter runs: "......the cine people who produce such movies do not care what effect they have on young minds—they only want money. If the cine people are mindless the fact that Doordarshan, a Government agency, telecast the movie, is example enough of how much it has degenerated...". Another letter on the same day runs: "Doordarshan is hell bent on spoiling our youngsters by screening such filthy movies which breed only vulgarity". The concerned picture mainly advocates premarital promiscuous sexual relations among the youths and adolescents and the Madras Doordarshan encourages such themes by telecasting them. There are many Tamil motion pictures, produced on perverted sex themes and the Madras Doordarshan has telecasted them in the past in spite of certain protests from the public. Thus the movies and the Doordarshan become the biggest agencies for degenerating the Indian culture and directing the youths and adolescents in the wrong direction in the name of entertainment. The consequences are premarital, permissive and promiscuous sexual relations which in turn lead to the breeding more AIDS cases and drug abuses. At this context, when the two most powerful mass media are imbibing perverting ideas in the minds of the youths not the duty of the Government to protect them from the greatest disaster they are facing today?

The sexually transmitted disease (STD) the AIDS is not a sudden emergence in some of the States in India nor it is imported in one day at one of the ports in India and distributed to various States. The ground in India, particularly in Maharashtra and Tamil Nadu was already fully fertilized for the germination of the AIDS. Otherwise, how there could be thousands of AIDS cases in these two States? We do not know exactly whether the premarital permissive and promiscuous sex themes of the movies of the past two decades had the influencing effect upon the youths' behaviour had created a fertile soil for the emergence of the AIDS or poverty and circumstances forced the young girls to go into the prostitutions where the girls had contracted the HI virus and transmitted to the males with whom they had sexual relations had caused the AIDS. Whatever the cause behind the emergence of the AIDS it has to be explored scientifically and preventive measures should be taken. Medical approach is to cure the disease and the psychological approach is to prevent it. Prevention is better than cure.

Glenn and Weaver (1979) state : "Survey research indicates that permissive attitudes about such activities as premarital sexual activity are more likely to be held by those with the most education. The effect across generations is more striking, with younger individuals expressing much more permissive attitudes than older ones". Survey studies provides evidence that the educated youths who are prone to premarital sexual relations are more easily accessible to the AIDS.

The AIDS is caused by the human sexual activities which are perverted and promiscuous in type. Therefore, it should be handled very carefully without hurting the feelings of normal and healthy human beings. Since the AIDS is a disease it should not be construed as purely a medical problem. The main aim of the preventive measure is to change the attitudes and behaviour of the people towards the premarital/permissive/promiscuous sexual activities. Sex is a feeling and cognitive aspect of human behaviour and it fulfils the biological needs. Since it is very sensitive in nature it should be psychologically dealt with. The approach is to create a sense of disgust or aversion for illegitimate and promiscuous sexual activities through acceptable methods. The risk-groups should be made to realize that such an act is wrong from health, moral and cultural points of view.

The serious consequences of the AIDS and the drug abuses should be presented to the risk-groups in attention-getting attractive manner and the risk-groups should be exposed to such publicities directly with all seriousness with the strong determination of changing their attitudes and behaviour pattern. This is not easy, but the success depends upon the psychological strategy. Why was the Family Planning and Birth Control programme of the Government of India not successful? The progress of the programme remained with some slogans and some birth control operations. It was not well conceived and planned. The population problem in our country was treated as the medical problem and, therefore, the whole responsibility was left with the medical professionals. Fawcatt (1970) one of the exponents of population research states that population is made up of people, and psychology is the study of people. The population growth is psycho-social-demographic problem. Therefore, there should be interdisciplinary approach to deal with it.

Before launching any nation-wide programme, it is important to know the attitudes of the people towards the problem to be tackled. Hence a preliminary study should be planned first of all to know the attitudes of the risk-groups towards the AIDS and the drug abuses and the causative factors like the various types of sexual relations and the effects of drug abuses. This type of primary study may throw some light upon the views held by the risk-groups about the AIDS and drug abuse. Launching any remedial measures directly upon these types of psycho-social problems will not result in alleviating the problems, because we may not be knowing correctly the nature of the problem prevailing at that time.

Cultural Approach

India is a nation of multiplicity of races, religions, cultures, castes and communities. But there was always unity in diversity and the

Indian cultural and social life were built upon the strong restrictive principles and any attempt to break away from them met with serious consequences. People in India for long time have been trying to uphold the cultural values. The cultural values were part of the social life till very recently, in solving everyday problems. The ancient Indian scientists had invincible faith in the cultural values. We need not miss the recent scientific developments in dealing the AIDS virus. Let us make best use of them as and when they are available for our purpose. The Indian ways of tackling deadliest disease may be used as the supplementary treatments and as the preventive measures as far as possible. Suresh (1991) states that the health authorities in India believe that the Acquired Immune-deficiency Syndrome (AIDS) could be controlled by the ancient yogic practices. There are certain sophisticated yogic practices which may protect our men and women from the AIDS. But what is required is to create a favourable and congenial atmosphere towards our ancient cultural heritage and wisdom. The values and the effectiveness of the yogic practices should be made available to everybody easily and it should be presented in attractive manner to the concerned population (risk-groups) and arouse their sensitivity towards the effectiveness of the yogic practices.

The Indian cultural heritage with special reference to the yogic practices should be made as a part of National Programme right from secondary education level to college level. Venkoba Rao (1990) states that the AIDS can be controlled by proper health education. The programme may be a part of physical education and should function as a curriculum of study. Or it may function as a separate department with varied health subjects. The programme need not be only with demonstrations of yogic practices, but also should combine lecture classes and examinations. Textbooks on this should be available easily everywhere. The syllabus should be devised on the basis of the essence of the Indian cultural heritage with special reference to yogic practices which should be associated with serious and deadliest diseases. There is no harm even if the same educational system continued at all levels (B.A., B.Sc., etc.) in all Indian Universities. If the programme is properly planned and sincerely implemented for a period of five years then it will have tremendous effect upon the health practices of our society. It may also promote discipline among the student community, a sense of self-development, self-confidence, and national feelings etc. The yogic practices of education should not be made as one of the money making professions nor a department which can provide jobs for the unemployed persons. It should be a service oriented National Programme with the view of promoting the Health of the Nation.

Any programme whether it is at national level or State level should be implemented with all seriousness and sincerity. First of all it is very important to know the trend prevailing in the concerned population or group which is considered as risk-group. We cannot teach new tricks to old. Therefore, the population we choose for programme should be amenable. The adolescent and the youth groups that we find in the Secondary, Higher Secondary schools and colleges seem to be the most suitable for this purpose. Since the aim is to protect our people from the infection of the HI virus and drug addiction, it is important to know what kind of information the adolescent and the youth population had imbibed about the AIDS and about the drugs that play disastrous role in the life of the victims.

The variables KAP may be quite suitable for this type of study. The 'K' stands for knowledge, that is the information about the infectious disease of the AIDS, the important causes and the consequences of it. 'A' stands for attitudes the people have developed towards the variables like, sex, heterosexual activities, type of sexual partners, prostitutes, sex education, the AIDS and the HI virus, drugs, drug addiction, heroin (white sugar), smoking of the drugs, intravenous injection, blood transfusion, the effects of heroin etc. 'P' stands for the practice of preventive measures for AIDS and drug addiction.

The preventive measures include all the precautionary measures like learning and acquiring correct knowledge about the diseases and avoiding situations causing diseases, educating people who are not aware of the diseases and their consequences and making them to get rid of such atmosphere. It may also include explaining the type of sufferings the human kind would face as the result of negligence of hygienic way of life. People all know that prevention is better than cure. Therefore, if the horrors of the dreaded disease are explained through suitable media and authoritative channels then it is possible to convince people and make them to accept the ideas relating to the AIDS and the drugs and drug addiction. Studies show that psychological methods and tools contribute to greater understanding of the prevailing and acute problems. Once if the people's attention is drawn towards the problem, then there would not be any difficulty in making them to think and realize the subsequent evils they might face consequent of their socially unacceptable activities.

The preventive measures should not be entrusted only with the research organizations and the core-groups. All the service oriented organizations and voluntary groups should come forward to share the responsibility with the Government in implementing the programme successfully.

ADOLESCENTS AND THE DRUG ABUSES

The population most suitable to study the AIDS and the drug abuses may be the adolescents who are supposed to be the risk-groups. Though it is important that all the adolescents studying in schools and colleges and the youths who are unemployed should be included in this study, a primary study may be limited only to the area where the AIDS is suspected to be spreading and the AIDS cases are prevalent, and drug abuses are rampant. Ten per cent of the sample from the adolescents and youths may be selected for this study. Generally the concept 'Adolescence' is associated with teen agers. Roughly it begins with some stage of sexual maturity. It is very difficult to decide its termination. It is presumed that adolescence ends when the individual attains some aspects of adult status. That is, when he is regarded as an adult in the eyes of law, in the eyes of his family members and his associates.

According to McCandless (1970) an adult is a person who must have the ability and willingness to make his own major decisions and he must have also the power to implement those decisions. If he can initiate practical steps to carry out the decisions then he is an adult, no matter what his age is. Liebert and other (1974) say that there is no clear boundary of years to define adolescence, though generally, the period may be said to begin with puberty, the onset of physical maturation (12 to 14 years of age) and to terminate where the individual assumes adult-like responsibilities such as marriage, full-time employment or a serious commitment to career training, usually between the ages of 18 to 20 years in U.S.A. culture. In Indian culture there is no definite age range of the adolescent period acceptable throughout the nation. Stott (1974) has stated that the adolescent period of development as all other human development periods is a time transition, of moving along a continuum from one signal point to the next. According to Stott the onset of puberty which usually occurs between the ages of 10 and 13 which is early adolescence, the middle adolescence occurs between the ages of 12 and 15 years and the later adolescence occurs between the ages of 16 and 20 years. But the age of adolescence varies from culture to culture. The three views expressed by the authors are from the developmental point of view.

This classification varies from the popular views to some extent. According to the Oxford English Dictionary, the adolescent's age ranges from 14 to 25 years for males and 12 to 21 years for females. It seems that there is no universally accepted age range for the adolescence. Till boys and girls move into adulthood they are adolescents only. Therefore, for the purpose of the study of the AIDS and the drug addiction the age of adolescents may be from 14 to 25 years as this age range seems to include early youthhood and appears to be rationale from several points of view in the Indian context. This is because, at the age of 14 the boys and girls enter the 10th standard or S.S.L.C and this is supposed to be the school final and the students leave the high school and enter higher secondary school at the age of 15. After having spent two years in the higher secondary school the students enter the college at the age of 17 in the first year of the Degree course. It takes 3 years for a student to complete the Degree course and another 2 years to complete the Post-graduate course. By this time the boy or girl completes 22 or 23 years. The same number of years is spent by a student in the professional Degree course also, such as Engineering, Medicine, Agriculture etc., unless one fails to get through the course successfully within the duration of the course. Some students complete their College or University course at the age of 24 or 25. Therefore, till one completes the college or University course he/she is an adolescent as he/she is believed to be living with adolescent habits and has not reached the stage of holding the adult's responsibilities. Therefore, the adolescent's age range from 14 to 25 years is quite acceptable as the type of classification encompasses also the early youth period.

It is observed that researches on AIDS often associate drug addiction with the AIDS. They state that more than 50 per cent of the drug addicts were found to be infected with HI virus as they often resort to intravenous drug injection through uncleaned syringes and needles and, therefore, drug addiction becomes one of the important causes of the AIDS. But it appears that the AIDS control team has not taken this aspect into confidence. Therefore, it is better that any study on AIDS should associate always the drug addiction with it.

The activists on one side try to reform society by all possible means with all their might. On the other side the delinquents strike out vigorously against it. When the delinquent gangs are induced to give up their active and violent search for kicks, they turn to drugs which they consider as the more effective substitute. Drug abuse among the adolescents has become more widespread during the past fifteen years in our country.

Coleman and Broen (1974) have observed that of the various substances associated with drug addiction, the hallucinogens (marijuana and LSDO), deliriants (air plane glue, aerosol sprays), and depressents (barbiturates), stimulants (cocaine) and opiates (heroin and morphine) are most widely and frequently used by the adolescents. Wolk (1969) has stated that the older adolescents were more familiar with hallucinogens especially marijuana and opiates. According to Akers (1970) there are variations on the basis of social-class and opiates and stimulants were more frequent among the adolescents from lower socio-economic classes. Psychologists who studied this problem have stressed a variety of general factors that may be at work. From the studies made by Vincent (1969) and Keeler (1968) it is known that the most common reasons the adolescents state for taking drugs like marijuana, heroin and morphine are curiosity-seeking, peer group conformity or social acceptance, tension relief, thought stimulation, the thrill or experiencing a psychotic-like state and unhappy home life. Thus we can see how the present day adolescents live in a culture using the word 'drug' and relies strongly on drugs and chemicals to eliminate their distress. A special pill for every ill and all purpose pill for any ills seem to be the philosophy of life of the adolescents.

The adolescent may develop more curiosity on the drugs that are well publicized and he is highly tempted to taste these drugs secretly and to experience the effects of them in solitude and sometimes in the company of the peers. When he finds the effects of the drugs highly exciting and intoxicating, freeing him from misery he wishes to use the drugs again and again and have the exciting experience. Thus one becomes drug abuse or dependence.

The practice of using the drugs is increasing day by day in India and it is becoming one of the most striking social changes to occur in 1980s, and the young people are the primary users of them in various ways. Much concern is expressed about the drug use by the leaders of various sections of societies and it causes anxieties to educationalists as it is becoming a serious problem for discipline and morale. It is also becoming a threat of possible physical damage. Psychological dependency and crime levels increase. The complicated issues surrounding drug abuse are not easy to resolve. This is only the beginning of a scientific study with the views of understanding some of the facts underlying the problem such as who are the main drug abusers and under what circumstances.

There are many different kinds of drugs that are consumed and they differ dramatically in composition and effects. Any one drug may vary in potency depending upon its dosage, quality and even individual's reaction to it. It difficult to obtain information about drug use as individuals choose not to share the experience they have had with illegal substances. With regard to the effects of marijuana it is considered to be more important among the drugs.

Goode (1970) has stated that there were two studies, conducted independently in New York City which showed that most of the drug users were in their late teens or early twenties. Nietzel and others (1970) also have observed that there were more men than women involved in all aspects of the drug culture—from testing to regular usage and to selling. However the chances were that the users irrespective of sex, were urban dwellers or people who live near the urban environment and they were all college youths. It was found that approximately 6 per cent of college students were drug users in 1966-67 in United States. There was striking increase in the percentage of college students who were using drugs in 1974. This increase was approximately twenty-five per cent.

If a systematic study is conducted in India among the adolescents and youths who are in schools and colleges there is a possibility of getting wonderful results on drug addiction and also some new results about the AIDS and the infectious HI virus. It is observed that the narcotic drugs are in regular usage and distribution in some parts of Tamil Nadu among the adolescents and youths. The Narcotic Control Bureau of Chennai often ceases brown sugar from the carriers. A systematic survey may be planned and conducted in certain districts of Tamil Nadu where the narcotic drugs are in usage. These districts are Thanjavur, Tiruchirapalli, Madurai, South Arcot, North Arcot and Chengulpattu. In these districts there are more HI virus infected cases, more cases of drug abuses and distribution of narcotic drugs. The adolescents in these districts are believed to be in practice of using drugs more than other districts except Chennai City. A separate study programme may be planned for Chennai City.

If possible the survey may be extended to all other districts of Tamil Nadu and to other risk-groups like the unemployed youths, bus drivers and conductors, auto-rickshaw drivers, certain section of movie stars, film technicians, industrial workers and policemen apart from the adolescents in schools and colleges. Opinions and attitudes may be elicited from these groups and other risk-groups to know what these groups actually feel and think about the AIDS, HI virus infection, sexually transmitted diseases, drug addiction and intravenous drug injection. Strategies of preventive measures may be worked out on the basis of these informations. This approach may facilitate to evolve correct preventive measures, particularly in finding out ways and means of changing the attitudes and behaviour of risk-groups towards the AIDS and drugs.

2

AIDS and Other Infectious Diseases

M. RAJAMANICKAM

INTRODUCTION

The scientific advancements are mostly based upon testing competing hypotheses to account for the observations for which immediate correct answers are not available. New methods of research in various disciplines bring out several new results and also make it possible to solve the problems untraced previously. The researches made by generations of scientists brought out many things for human comforts and discomforts.

The physical and chemical sciences are mainly concerned with the properties of matter and energy and the relationships between them which included mechanistics, optical, electricity and magnetism, atomic and nuclear power and all possible products of natural resources and also concerned with the composition of properties and the reactions of substances. Biological sciences are concerned with organisms including their structure and functioning, evolution, distribution and the inter-relationships and also the structure and functions of a particular or a group of organisms.

The physiological psychology, a branch of psychology is concerned with the study and correlation of physiological and psychological events. The medical and chemical sciences are mainly concerned with discovery of medicines and methods of treatment of patients for those who are suffering from damning diseases, with drugs and remedies. Animal research models enabled the researchers to make hopeful progress that is found more important for the human behaviour problems in question.

But all the progresses, inventions and discoveries in these areas however were providing comforts, happiness, cure and remedies there are certain uncontrolled forces causing great harms which man could never imagine. There were unexpected and uncontrolled natural forces like earthquake, storms or tempest, floods, famine resulting in killing millions of people in the past and also occurring periodically even in the present times. All the scientific and technological advancements, inventions and discoveries were found helpless against these natural calamities. Apart from these uncontrolled natural forces, there were also dangerous epidemic diseases periodically killing millions of people. Man with all his intellectual skills and talents could not produce any permanent remedies against these forces. The history of human race has witnessed many such events.

There are still many gaps, discrepancies, and mysteries in our present knowledge of scientific explorations. The unresolved mysterious icon points to some of these problems can be thought of for only future research in various disciplines.

The human surroundings are day by day becoming highly congested, polluted and contaminated with infectious materials which spoil the living areas with all sorts of poisonous materials. As a result of these, there are ample chances for the development of bacteria, viruses, pathogenetic microorganisms. Since these are developing in human living environment human beings get easily infected by these disease causing viruses or microorganisms. Since people neglect hygienic way of life and do not learn to live hygienically, poisonous insects of various types are produced in the garbage collected living areas. As a result of these some kind of infectious diseases attack all living creatures and man is the most affected living creature. The human body is not an anti-infectious.

The most important threat to human beings is the environmental pollutions from liquid and wastage or garbage collections from which infectious germs and insects are generated everyday. The three important basic materials components which are essential for living are the land, water and air. When pollution takes place in these, there is no healthy life for man. Several types of infectious diseases are caused because of this condition and man is helpless except to suffer from all these.

The bacteria or the viruses invade the human body and get into the brain and damage the brain and nerve cells. All the infectious diseases are easily communicable and can spread out. Apart from the epidemic diseases, the infectious diseases were also causing serious consequences and deaths. Some of the important infectious diseases the human beings are facing are the tuberculosis, pneumonia, cancer, typhoid, yellow fever and typhus.

TUBERCULOSIS

This is a severe communicable infectious disease, characterized by the formation of *tubercle*. It is caused by tubercle-bacillus which is most frequently affecting the lungs. It may affect one or both lungs. Sometimes any inside bodily parts may be affected. It is also called pulmonary consumption, which is the tuberculosis of the lymphatic glands. The chronic asthma in many cases develops into tuberculosis.

PNEUMONIA

Pneumonia is a highly infections disease. This also infects the lungs. Sometimes both lungs get infected with pneumonia. In this state the air sacs (alveoli), ponch-like parts in the lungs become filled with liquid which renders them useless for breathing. The person who is infected with this disease find it very difficult to breathe. It is usually caused by the bacteria especially the *pneumo coccal* or viral infections. It mainly causes inflammation in lungs or produces inflammatory substances in the lungs. One or both lungs are affected by *bacillus coccus* – microbe pneumococcus. In most of the cases it develops from chronic asthma. The treatment for this is quite similar to tuberculosis, because the disease attacks the lungs.

CANCER

Cancer is any type of malignant growth or tumour caused by abnormal and uncontrolled cell division which may spread out through the lymphatic system or blood stream to any bodily parts. The diseased brain tumour cells are transmitted to lungs and through which to other parts of the body and cause serious consequences. People suffer from cancer in various parts of the body. Though the main bodily part for cancer is lungs, the other parts of the body like the mouth, nose, prostate in the case of man, and breast, uterus in the case of women are attacked. No part of human body is spared from the attack of cancer. Cancer is also caused in the eyes, throat and also in blood, which is called blood cancer. Some people die of blood cancer.

Apart from the cause of cell division for the cause of cancer, there are also psychological causes for cancer. Stress and emotions influence cancer. There are strong links between emotions and cancer. Greer (1983) in his studies observed the psychological influences on the cause and outcome of cancer. In another study he observed depression and the feelings of helplessness have been found associated with cancer. Greer states that breast cancer was the cause of life-long suppression of anger. Smoking and tobacco chewing also cause cancer. Ultimately cancer drives human beings to psychogenic behaviour and the person dies down out of cancer.

YELLOW FEVER

This is an acute infectious disease of tropical and sub-tropical climatic conditions, characterized by fever, hemorrhages, vomiting of blood and jaundice, it is caused by a virus, transmitted by the bite of a female mosquito of the species *Aedes aegyptie*. This disease is also called *Yellow Jack* and *Black Vomit*. It is controlled by immunization and by avoiding mosquitoes.

TYPHOID

Typhoid is always associated with fever. Typhoid is an acute infectious disease characterized by high fever, rose-coloured spots in the chest, or abdomen, abdominal pain and occasional intestinal bleedings. This disease is caused by *bacillus salmonalls typhosa* and also when persons ingested with contaminated food and water. Typhoid is also called enteric fever. It is also caused by the contact of waste matter excreted by the infectious human beings.

TYPHUS

Typhus is one of the groups of acute infectious *rickettsial* diseases transmitted by fleas, lice etc., characterized by high fever, skin rash and severe headache. Typhus is of three types. They are (1) Epidemic typhus, (2) Murine typhus, and (3) Brill's disease. The first two are found world over and the last one prevails in the East Coast of U.S.A. It is mostly caused by flea which is a small wingless jumping insect. It is a blood sucking parasite.

These acute infectious diseases prevail all over the world and human beings suffer from these diseases. In serious cases people die with all medicines and methods of treatment. If man escaped from the epidemic diseases by administering the medicines and treatment he discovered, he cannot escape easily from the infectious diseases of some kind.

OTHER INFECTIOUS DISEASES

Researches in the fields of medicine, chemical sciences and physiology are going on as non-stopping process and now and then new hopeful results are brought for vitalizing human body and mind. A new science had emerged with the view of fulfilling the gaps and deficiencies in human endeavours of the past. It is the biological psychology which deals with both mind and body. Biological psychology is mainly based upon certain hypotheses formulated with regard to the brain infections. It is whether human experiences could increase the mental capacity still better or make it for super function of the brain for solving the emerging pathogenic and psychogenic problems human beings are now and then facing.

Biological scientists explore the bodily basis of human experience and behaviour. They are also interested in the ways in which the bodily states and the processes could produce and control behaviour and cognition and the way in which behaviour and cognition in turn influence the bodily system. Many scientific inventions and discoveries have contributed to this scheme. But still there is wide gap and discrepancies to be fulfilled by the present generation of scientists to the posterity. Therefore, if we are really interested in finding out the correct solution for the existing problems, we must keep ourselves seriously in multiphase research work involving disciplines such as psychology, anatomy, biochemistry, endrocriology, genetics, neurology, psychology, psychopharmacology and zoology. In order to have a very wide view in all directions we must try to rise above the limits of any one of the single discipline.

Man is constantly striving hard to get rid of the uncontrolled fatal diseases which are highly infectious. There are severe infectious diseases other than we have discussed earlier. These infectious diseases cause panic among the people. Generally infection means the invasion or forcible entry of the virus or bacteria into the body. The virus is forcibly entering the body. It is the disease producing microorganism (pathogenic). The central nervous system, the brain is invaded by a wide variety of infectious agents such as virus, bacteria, fungi, and metazoan parasites. The diagnosis and the treatment for the infection are important aspects of chemical observation. Therefore, the infections of the nervous system spread out quickly from the infection to various parts of the body such as the ears, nose and throat (ENT). The virus may also enter directly into the brain, because of head injury and skull fractures. Infections of the nervous system (glial cells) are very serious as the affected nervous and glial cells are destroyed. There are a number of ways by which infections destroy the neural cells.

The important symptoms of the infections are lowered blood pressure and other symptoms in blood circulations, fever, general malaise, headache and delirium. There are two main types of infectious diseases of the brain, apart from the infectious diseases discussed above. They are: (1) Cerebral Syphilis, (2) Epidemic

Encephalitis. Syphilis is an infectious disease caused by the microorganisms, treponema pallidum. Pusey (1933) has stated that syphilis is an infectious disease that has played an important role in the lives and happiness of human beings and was the cause of innumerable number of lives all over the world.

The reason for such disastrous consequences is that the syphilis is a sexually transmitted disease. It is an infectious venereal disease, easily and rapidly spreads out.

Syphilis may be defined as a venereal disease caused by infection with the microorganism *Treponema Pallium*, which is characterized by an ulcerating chancre usually on the external genital and progressing through the lymphatic system to nearly all tissues of the body, producing serious clinical manifestations.

Syphilis, according to experts is as old as mankind. But it is dealt with in various ways and existed in different names. The common name given to this is venereal disease which is transmitted in sexual intercourse. The 'treponema pallidum' invades the human body through mucus membrane after being contracted either during sexual intercourse or through oral or genital relations. Syphilis may be also transmitted by an infected women to her child.

This disease may show its first indication by a small sore in the area of the infected lips, genitals or anus. This symptom may appear after three weeks. This is also called general paresis or brain syphilis. This disease was spread out in Europe during last quarter of fifteenth century and was named as *Great pox*. It was also called by some other names. In the first quarter of nineteenth century it was called as *general paralysis*.

All these diseases are caused by infections of some types. There are several types of infections that affect the central nervous system, the brain. Mainly there are four types of infections. They are: (a) Viral infections, (b) Bacterial infections, (c) Mycotic infections, and (d) Parasite infections.

(a) The infections caused by viruses mainly attack the brain. The viruses are of any groups of microscopic entities which consists of a single nucleic acid which is multiplying within the cell and most of them are psychogenic in nature and cause diseases. Some viruses are called neurotropic viruses which have strong attraction for the central nervous system i.e. the brain, and cause injury in the whole area of the brain. This makes the brain bodily damaged.

(b) The bacterial infections are caused by a large group of microorganisms which are called bacteria. The important characteristics of these bacteria are producing diseases. The disease in the central nervous system is caused through blood streams. The most common disorders the bacterial infections causing are the meningitis and brain abscesses. The abscesses produce bacteria which cause death of cells in the affected area.

(c) The Mycotic infections are caused by fungus by entering into the brain. The brain strongly resists this infection. But, however fungi invades the brain when the resistance becomes weak due to other diseases like the pneumonia or tuberculosis.

(d) The parasitic infections produce amebiasis and malaria. The parasitic infections invade the brain and cause severe diseases. Amebiasis is caused by infection of the protozoan ameba which results in encephalitis and brain abscesses. Malaria is caused by *protozoa* of the *genus plasmodium* which are transmitted by infectious mosquitoes. The cerebral malaria is also caused by these mosquitoes.

Cerebral Infections

The micro-organisms like the viruses, bacteria and fungi get into the body and infect the brain. These infections almost get into the brain and damage the brain and nervous tissues. There are mainly two types of infectious diseases caused in the brain. These are cerebral syphilis and epidemic encephalitis.

Cerebral Syphilis

The brain is connected with almost all mental disorders. Since the brain cells are damaged or destroyed, by the infections, brain functions are affected and behaviour disorders or organic psychoses are taking place. Syphilis is an infectious disease caused by the microorganisms called *Treponema Pallidum.* Treponema pallidum is an animal microorganism named *spirochoeta* which causes syphilis.

Cerebral syphilis has a long history right from the time of fifteenth century onwards. It does not mean that it did not exist before that period. There are also references in the medieval literature and history. Girrolamo Francastore (1483-1553) an Italian physician, astronomer and a poet in the city of Verona wrote a poem in which he used the name of this disease, syphilis. The poem itself was named as Syphilis. The poetic incidents were based upon the analogy of Aeneas, Thebais etc., the Trojan Princes. The poet, Francastore had described the adventurous activities of these princes. In the poem a character named Shepherd Syphilus was the first victim of this disease. The Trojans were the original intalitants of the Ancient Troy. Syphilis was studied in detail by a quite number of scholars and provided with interesting information.

Kemble (1936) had stated that syphilis was first traced in West Indies. It was Columbus (1451-1506) an Italian navigator and an explorer in the service of Spain had discovered the New World in 1492. He first landed in West Indies with his sailors in 1492. During his stay in West Indies, his sailors has sexual contact with West Indies women and got infected with the syphilis and they brought it to Europe. Kemble stated that Columbus himself had contracted this disease and it had become very severe when he had the second voyage in 1494 to West Indies and the symptoms of syphilis appeared in him. When Columbus had made the third voyage in 1498 he had the severe attack of syphilis and died of it in 1506. There is legal holiday in most of the States in U.S., on December 12th 1492, the day Columbus landed in West Indies.

Cerebral Syphilis, thus had played a disastrous role in the lives and happiness of the people in the past. The present century is witnessing still much greater dangerous situation through syphilis and exactly quite similar disease, the AIDS. It prevails with all its strength because of our social and cultural norms are relaxed to the maximum possible and by accepting the premarital permissive promiscuous sexual activities and considering the obscene as fashion. Pusey (1933) while writing about syphilis has stated that it has killed millions of people all over the world in the past centuries. Persons who were infected with syphilis do not wish to reveal it out of shame and modesty. The most important reason is that it is an infectious disease rooted in human sex life and it in a sexually transmitted disease.

Another similar disease with which human being suffer from is the *Gonorrhea*. This is also an infectious disease sexually transmitted. This disease is causing the same type of suffering as syphilis. Gonorrhea may be defined as an infectious venereal disease caused by a virus called *gonococcus*. This is characterized by burning sensation while unrinating in the case of males and in the case of females it causes *mucopurulent discharge* from the urethra or vagina.

TYPES OF SYPHILETIC SYNDROMES

The syphiletic brain infections have three different syndromes. They are: (1) General paresis, (2) Juvenile paresis, and (3) Meningovascular syphilis.

General Paresis

The general paresis is the loss of physical and mental abilities. It is caused due to brain damage. Syphilis generally causes the brain disease. General paresis is stated as the mental disease caused by the syphilatic infection of the brain. This disease or disorder is also known as *general parlalytic.* The syphilis virus is called *spirochaeta* which enters into the brain step by step and destroys the brain tissues. The syphiletic infection takes long time to make its appearance as it slowly destroys the brain cells. At this stage immediate treatment should be given, otherwise it causes death.

Clinical observations state that general paresis is a paralysis of motor functions, which mainly affect the voluntary movements of the bodily parts. Syphilis is the disease of the central nervous system. It is also called demontia paralytic. If treatment is not given to syphilis for two or three years, it develops into general paresis,

paresis, which may result in the death of the pèrson. General paresis develops in human at the age of forty and above. Ford (1970) and Strange (1971) have stated that syphilis cases increased rapidly in United States and in the year 1970 alone there were one million persons suffering from syphilis and they were not given treatment. In developing countries the number of persons suffering from syphilis is still greater and they were left out unnoticed. The behavioural symptoms of syphilis vary widely. There is a general lack of cognitive and feeling aspects and the person is very much interested is promiscuous sexual activities.

Persons who suffer from the general paresis of syphilis do not care for anything in the early period. Since they are young they do not bother about the consequences of this disease. But when the disease has advanced many physical and mental symptoms appear. The person's eyesight is very much affected and there will be speech disorder, and loss of memory. The syphilatic patient of general paresis at this stage may be involved in all sorts of anti-social activities. When the disease becomes still advanced the patient meets with death.

General paresis is of three types such as the expensive type, depressed type and demanded type. *The expensive* type of general paresis patients always make overestimation about themselves. These patients claim that they are extremely well and also say that they are worth millions. They mostly live on delusions and hallucinations. *The depressed type* of patients behave like organic psychotic patients. These patients to some extent realize of their failures to reach to the life situations. They often develop fantastic delusions. They accept that they lost their brain and develop a tendency to commit suicide and die. They develop extreme anxiety and depression.

The Demanded Type of general paresis patients step by step are deteriorating in their personality and in the intellectual functions. They suffer from loss of memory and personality disorder. They will be experiencing simple type of delusions and hallucinations.

Juvenile Paresis

This is a common mental disorder prevailing in many countries. Mostly in developing countries this is a common disease which occurs in childhood and in adolescent periods. This is often accompanied by mental and physical disorders. These patients generally suffer from loss of memory, speech disorder and malfunctions of motor activities. In Parran's (1987) study it was observed that more than half of the children were blind at birth due to syphilis in the family. Further many children in such families die in the first week itself.

Meningovascular Paresis

Syphilis of this type is somewhat different from other types of syphilis. Meninges consisted of three protective sheets of tissues that surround the brain and spinal cord called, the *duramaten* mater *piamater* and *arachnoid.* They are the membranes, soft thin layers covering the brain and spinal cord, which is infected by a virus called *meningitis*. The syphiletic viruses damage the blood vessels and the meninges of the brain and also cause disorders. The symptoms of this type of syphilis vary from the general paresis. The symptoms of this meningo-vascular paresis are mainly continuous or severe headache, giddiness, fever, stiffneck, rapid pulse and respiration, eye defect and speech disorder. This paresis is also called cerebral syphilis. This syphilis spreads out more rapidly than the other forms.

Treatment

This disease mainly attacks the brain and, therefore, all types of syphiletic diseases should be attended only by a medical specialist. The syphilitic infection should be attended immediately. Delay in the treatment may result in the damage of the brain and the brain tissues would be destroyed. Because the syphiletic infection quickly reaches the brain, once this takes place any type of treatment will have very little effect. But the invention of penicillin and other anti-biotic medicines made dramatic effect on syphilis and syphiletic patients who were relieved from the fatal consequences.

The role played by the syphilis is in no way smaller than the disastrous consequences caused in the past and causing now by the AIDS. The American Medical Association (1969) has given an alarming statistical figure about the rapid increase of syphiletic cases all over the world. Subsequently, Fleming *et al.*, (1970) have published a statistics that there was an increase of more than two million new cases of syphilis every year in the United States alone during 1960 and 1970. Since it is sexually transmitted disease persons who were infected with this disease did not seek treatment soon after the infection out of sense of shame. They sought the treatment when it had become severe by damaging the brain tissues.

Treatment to juvenile paresis is almost the same as given to the general paresis. However, the child is innocent he/she has to suffer from the syphilis because of his/her mother. Women who had the syphilis are likely to infect the developing children in their stomachs and the children will be born with the infection of the syphilis. These children are said to be having the *congenital syphilis*. This type of syphilis could have avoided if the pregnant women had taken the treatment during the period of pregnancy.

All the syphletic diseases discussed above are cerebral syphilis in the sense that they all attack the central nervous system, the brain and cause disorders. Further all these diseases are also associated with virus or bacterial infections. But the infections are of different types and hence the treatments also vary with infection. It has been experienced that the virus infections are extremely difficult to treat. There are no drugs that could counteract or neutralize the effects of the poisonous infection. But the only way is to allow the disease to have its own course. Kolb and Wishew (1990) are of the view that the cerebral infections by the virus or bacteria are treated with antibiotic drugs. Antibiotic drugs are often used in the treatments of this type of diseases.

Epidemic Encephalitis

Epidemic encephalitis is also an acute infectious disease caused by virus. Specifically encephalitis is a disease of inflammation of the brain tissues caused by a number of agents, mostly the viruses carried by insects. The epidemic encephalitis is the disease of the central nervous system caused by infilterable viruses. In the earlier days this disease is called the inflammation of the brain, caused by viruses. This disease was identified only after the First World War in Europe and in America. This disease is mostly found among children and young adults. It is now widely prevalent in developing countries in Asia and Africa. Bad cold and flu are the most commonly appearing symptoms in the early stage. In the advanced stage the symptoms are fever, drowsiness and stupor. The person who suffers from this disease is often very lethargic and is found all the times sleeping. One of the important symptoms found in the patient of this disease is the paralysis of the eye muscles and the patient finds it very difficult to have a correct vision. It is because of this the patient becomes lethargic. This disease is also called *sleeping sickness*. When this disease gets a serious stage, the patient becomes emotionally excited, gets irritation and also agitated and violent. According to Coleman (1975) the effects of this disease become very serious in children and in young adults. The children who were cheerful and well behaved earlier, become very impulsive, ruthless, destructive, homicidal and sexually deviant. These children should be immediately hospitalized, failing which may result in outrageous activities and meet with death in some forms.

In adult persons this disease in the after effect state becomes very acute and there are symptoms of Parkinson's syndrome. There may be also paralysis is some of the bodily parts. In the after effect of this disease there may be mostly headshaking and handshaking. The serious after effect of epidemic encephalitis is the stiffness of the muscles and jerking of arms. The patients may have breathing difficulties based upon the emotional excitements.

The epidemic encephalitis in the state of Parkinson's Syndrome, the mental symptoms are the loss of interest in life activities and inability to concentrate in work. The patient becomes very depressive, pessimistic and develops utter hatred for life and tries to commit suicide and die. The patient mostly lives on systematized delusions and this state mostly prevails after sixty years in men.

Treatment

The epidemic encephalitis, since is an infectious disease caused by the invading viruses and bacteria and the brain is mostly damaged, it can be attended and cured only by medical treatments. But an immediate attention can be made by administering some antibiotics which are believed to destroy the invading viruses and bacteria. But there are also some new techniques of drug therapies which are hoped to control the infections of the brain and nervous tissues. Experts believe that it is also possible to control this disease by some psychological and educational techniques in children and young adults.

These techniques are based upon mainly by adopting hygienic way of life, avoiding crowds, high risk groups, and by changing the beliefs and attitudes, avoiding provocative magazines and literature and educating the children and youths with cultural and social norms. They should be kept away from offensive or outrageous to accepted standards of decency and modesty.

SYPHILIS AND AIDS

The infectious disease, syphilis was carried from West Indies to Europe by Columbus and his sailors at the end of the fifteenth century. It was carried by men and not by women. But how it could spread out in the whole of Europe and England? The answer for this question in precise form could be that it is an infectious disease which could be sexually transmitted from an infected person, male or female, to an uninfected person male or female. Since it could spread out rapidly by sexual contacts, the infected sailors might have had sexual intercourse with uninfected women and the disease could have been transmitted. These infected women when they had sexual contacts with other man transmits the disease to him. This was how within a short time syphilis spread out in the whole of Europe. But some medical scientists differ from this view and state that Columbus and his sailors alone cannot be held responsible for this unhappy incidence.

Syphilis might have been already prevailing in Europe since it is a sexual disease. One possible hypothesis is that any person male or female who is having sexual activities frequently with multiple partners is likely to get infected with some kind of sexual disease. This hypothesis can be verified in any community and in any culture. The frequent multiple partnership in sex activities may transmit some disease bacteria to an uninfected person. Further, a particular culture might have been immuned to some kind of germs or bacteria and when this body come into contact with another body of different culture which is not immunized to any kind of germs or bacteria may have their own effect. This effect may be syphilis or gonorrhea or even AIDS or any sexual disease.

Further, it is not possible to eliminate the cultural and racial factors. It is true that some cultural groups may be living in very unhealthy places in unhygienic way, without any clean habits. In most of the big cities in India thousands of people live in slum areas where there are all sorts of animals living with them and the area would be full of stinking. The environment may be producing toxic germs and insects. People who live in such areas are immunized to such unhealthy way of life. These immunized people when come into contact with the people of other cultural and social set-up, there may be certainly some kind of bacterial transmission taking place which may be of some infectious disease and when the contact is of sexual type, the resulting effect may be of some kind of sexual disease.

There are also approved red-light areas in big cities like Kolkata and Mumbai. Visitors to such areas are likely to get infected with venereal diseases. Studies made on this issue bring to light that there are certain communities in India who take up prostitution as their profession and young girls even at the age 12 or 13 years are engaged in the profession of prostitution. Whatever income they make out of this they are satisfied. They are not bothered about the consequences of their activities. Sibnath Deb (2002) has presented a research paper about the pathetic life led by the commercial sex workers and their children in an International Conference held in New Zealand in 1998. Deb collected data from the red-light areas of North Kolkata. Deb states that there is no fixed time for their business. All the 24 hours are their business hours. Instead of stating them as prostitutes, Deb calls them as commercial sex workers. These commercial sex workers are having contacts with multiple partners every day. Therefore, there is every chance for the visitor to carry back some bacteria which may cause sex disease after a few days.

Generally persons who visit such commercial sex workers area do not reveal anything about the infection they had developed. The persons secretly take remedial measures and get rid of it. Only in very serious cases the matter is brought to light. Venereal disease has become quite common among the high risk groups. Syphilis is little advanced stage which may manifest with certain symptoms. At this stage it needs immediate attention, failing which it may result in death.

Syphilis was said to be existing in India. One of the evidences traced was in Vasco da Gama (1469-1524). Vasco da Gama was a Portuguese navigator who discovered the sea route from Portugal to India around the Cape of Good Hope and landed with his sailors in Goa, a small town in the West, coast in 1498. Vasco da Gama, when returned to Portugal, he and his sailors carried with them the venereal disease from Goa and spread it out in Portugal. There are also references in Tamil literature about the female diseases. There were women who were professionally engaged in promiscuous sexual activities. Rich men and the landlords used to adopt one or two such women as concubines and patronize them. In such instances there were incidences of venereal diseases. This practice was prevailing all over India and such women were called *devadasis*. They were existing in different names in different regions and they were permitted to have the promiscuous sexual activities with the men who desired to have sexual relationships. All these might have contributed to some kind of venereal or sex diseases. Therefore, we may state that though the sex disease was not prevailing in the name of syphilis in India in the past centuries, the sex disease was prevailing on some other names.

As human life is getting rapidly changing due to technological developments, man's sex life also is changing in varied ways. The change of human life style is deviating from normal root and different interpretations are given. Premarital permissive promiscuous sexual activities are becoming very common and they are justified. Varied explanations are given to aberrations. Sexual deviations, rape, adultery, child abuse are all justified by some means. Man never hesitates in the present times to commit any type of sexual crime as he can escape easily from the punishment. Mass media of communication, magazines, motion pictures, Television and all other media make it a fashion to produce obscene themes and display. All these irregularities no doubt contribute to the development of some kind of sex disease. The extreme styles in fashion result in producing high risk groups who become victims of all kinds of sex diseases which become serious social problems.

After Columbus had discovered the New lands, there were large number of Europeans migrating to America and they were badly in need of men to assist them and work in the fields. The African Negroes were easily available for them and one of the African countries sponsored with their men and women was Uganda. They were taken to America during the period of colonization and there was racial intermixture among the Europeans who migrated to America and the Negroes. The white Europeans who have settled in America might have had the sexual activities with the Negro women who were migrated from Uganda and other African countries. The migration, colonization and the racial intermixture were going on from the middle of sixteenth century onwards.

During the course of four hundred years (1550-1950) due to racial intermixture and sexual contact between the white Europeans in America and the Negroes, some kind of sex disease might have been infected. The American settlers thought that it might be some kind of venereal disease. But the Americans did not take cognizance of it in the beginning and did not give any importance to it. Only after 1950 when there were large number of deaths, the American had become suddenly awakened and started studying it deeply. The medical scientists after investigating it for a long time found that it is sexually transmitted disease, but not syphilis and something else. They have observed that this is sex infected disease, but very serious and dangerous than syphilis. If this is really sex infected disease it should not have emerged all of a sudden.

The medical scientists, were able to observe the difference between the sexually transmitted disease, the syphilis which was also killing large number of persons and the present situation in which large number of persons were killed within a very short period of its infection. They were of the view that some virus or bacteria which is more dangerous than the *Treponema Pallidum,* which was causing syphilis, must be the cause of this disease and they named it as Acquired Immune Deficiency Syndrome (AIDS). The specific virus, which was causing this disease, was diagnosed as Human Immunodeficiency Virus (HIV).

In tracing the root cause of the AIDS, one theory is that it was taken to America from Africa by the Uganda African Negroes when they were taken to America. The European settlers in America needed the services of these Negroes. The AIDS was prevalent among the green monkeys in Uganda and these monkeys might have bitten the Negroes or the Negroes might have eaten the flesh of these green monkeys and might have contracted this disease. In this way the disease was prevailing among the Negroes and when they migrated to America they carried it with them. The Americans when they had sexual contact with the Negro women, they had contracted this disease. If this theory is accepted as the root cause of the AIDS in America, AIDS should have emerged in America by the end of sixteenth or during seventeenth centuries and not in the middle of twentieth century after 1950s. Or they might have mistaken it for syphilis and taking treatments. Therefore, associating Uganda Negroes with the root cause of the AIDS among the Americans may be taken only as hypothetical.

Many researchers are still on the AIDS and reveal different views. Nurnberg (1984) had asserted the cause with HIV virus and not with psychological stressors. He stated that the AIDS patient faces to opportunistic neurological infections of *cytomegalovirus.* This view was not agreeable to the later researchers. Ho and his co-workers (1985) are of the view that the symptoms of the AIDS are characteristic of what is known as AIDS dementia complex (ADC). The HIV virus has the ability to cross the brain-blood-barrier, the defence mechanism of the brain, and damages the brain. Nurnberg confirms this view and states that though the patient is infected by the opportunistic neurological infections of cytomegalovirus, the HIV virus directly attacks the brain.

Syphilis as a venereal disease takes time for damaging the brain and nerve cells, but AIDS takes very little time to cause damage to the brain. Finally, both the diseases cause damage to the brain, behaviour disorder and also death. Researches are still at large with regard to the origin, functions and the consequences of the AIDS. Whether the AIDS is developed from syphilis of very serious type or developed out of some toxic substances got into the body and infected the blood to produce some kind of virus which gets into the semen and caused this disease. The chemical scientists produce various kinds of poisonous or toxic materials which infect the human body very seriously. These toxic materials are mixed in food and water and also made to smell, certain poisonous materials which all cause, it is said, psychotic disorders and death.

Since AIDS was found very recently, only after 1970 it must be a new development out of something which already existed and caused danger to human beings. Any harmful substance may get into the body blood and also brain and cause some serious disease and can kill humans. The terrorist organizations, of late manufactured some poisonous substance which is supposed to kill man at the very instance of smelling it. It is said that these materials are highly infectious. Similar material might have been manufactured for some purpose which might have infected human blood and through which it got into the human sex life. The terrorist organizations have recently released a poisonous and infectious substance called *Anthrax* and it is said, that they also manufactured still more powerful substances. If the researchers of the AIDS go into the origin and development of the HIV virus and find out from which substance this virus has developed and how it become infectious in human sexual activities, then the remedial measures might have become easy.

At present the name given to the virus which causes the AIDS is Human Immunodeficiency Virus. But this is only referring to the function of some virus, the virus that could weaken the immunity of the body. Any virus may weaken the immunity of the body. Then shall we assume that a virus that could weaken the immunity of the body can be called as HIV virus? It infers that the name of the AIDS causing virus is not yet correctly identified and explained. Therefore, we may also assume that some poisonous chemical substance manufactured by man must be the source of the origin of the virus which causes the AIDS. This hypothesis can be tested from the available materials, like the Anthrax. The available name of the virus, other than the HIV virus, is the cytomegalovirus.

One important reason for formulating this hypothesis is that the AIDS was brought to the attention of the world only after 1970. Before that it was syphilis that was causing psychotic disorders and causing deaths. The American Medical Association (1960) has stated that syphilis is rapidly increasing all over the world. Fleming has given the figures that there was an increase of more than two million cases of syphilis every year in America during 1960 and 1970. Blood samples were collected in America from all over the world in 1972 and were analysed to trace the root of the AIDS. The root was somewhat traced in 1979 from the Ugandian blood sample. From this result the American Medical experts were able to state that the root was among the Ugandian Negroes. But the Ugandians went to America during the period of colonization. It must have been in sixteenth or seventeenth century. If the Ugandians were infected with the HIV virus, it should have had its effect when they went to America in sixteenth or seventeenth century. But till 1980 it was believed that the infectious disease with which the American and others were suffering was syphilis. The HIV virus, according to Ho and his associates (1985) was from the *cerebrospinal fluid and neural tissues.*

By analyzing the available information critically, the infectious diseases, the AIDS, syphilis, and tuberculosis, we may find that these diseases have something in common. With regard to the symptoms, AIDS causes severe physiological consequences of painful feelings. The other symptoms are severe anxiety, depression, nervous tension, obsessive-compulsive neurosis and also all types of psychosomatic disorders. The symptoms of syphilis are, severe headaches, dizziness, unclear eyesight, lack of concentration, delirium, horrible sore and bone ulcers. The psychological symptoms are almost the same. Tuberculosis reveals the same symptoms as the syphilis and the AIDS. The treatment to tuberculosis and the AIDS in the beginning stage is the same. Coleman (1975) states that the syphilis for a long time was baffling the medical scientists and there was no specific name for it. It was simply stated as venereal disease. Each nation was blaming the other nation for its cause. The Mercenaries and the Adventurers of fifteenth and sixteenth centuries had contributed to the rapid spread of this disease. In the beginning the painful sufferings of syphilis were very severe. It was extremely contagious and unusually virulent. This disease attacked the persons in an outrageous manner.

This disease spread out in England during 1498. It was Vasco da Gama and his sailors were mainly responsible for this. This disease had an outbreak in 1498 in India and the Portuguese who were there carried it to their country and from there it spread out to England and to other countries. It also spread out to China in the beginning of sixteenth century. This disease received the specific name as *syphilis* only in 1530. This disease was conquered by the medical scientists only after four hundred years.

Looking into consequences and the violent outrageous attacks, the syphilis was spreading out during the course of four hundred years all over the world, we may state that this disease was found to be more dangerous than the AIDS that we are experiencing today. The discovery of the Penicillin and antibiotics medicines and treatment around 1950s were able to cure the syphilis. But at present suitable medicines and treatment for AIDS are yet to be discovered. Both the diseases are highly contagious and infectious and sexually transmitted. They attack human very violently and make them suffer both physically and mentally.

Diagnosis and Classification

Syphilis is clinically diagnosed as a general paresis. General paresis is a mental disorder and associated with syphilis of the brain. It is a highly infectious disease caused by the microorganism, called *treponema pallidum* which destroys the brain tissues. It is also called general paralysis. Since the brain tissues are destroyed by the infection of the virus, it is considered as the organic brain syndromes. Therefore, it is classified as one of the organic psychoses.

The AIDS is also a highly contagious and infectious disease and sexually transmitted. The HIV virus destroys the brain and nervous tissues. The destruction of any bodily parts by some infectious virus results in causing mental disorders. Therefore, the AIDS may be classified as one of the organic brain syndromes. Hence, AIDS in an organic psychosis. There was some difference of opinion regarding the classification of the AIDS. The reason is that most of the symptoms are quite similar to psychological stresses. Therefore, it was classified as one of the functional psychoses. Snider (1985) has challenged this view and strongly established that it is an organic mental syndrome since it is having the characteristics of the effects of the HIV virus. Further, some neurological complications also were observed in the AIDS patients. It is Nurnberg (1984) who has first stated, that it is an organic mental syndrome, on observing it in his patients. The symptoms are attributed to HIV virus and not to the psychological stresses. Nurnberg states that the HIV virus directly attacks the brain and destroys the brain tissues and causes the disease, the AIDS. It is also observed that the AIDS patients are infected with the *cytomegalovirus* and the disease is caused. The HIV virus directly attacks the central nervous system, the brain and destroys the brain tissues and causes the behaviour disorders or organic psychosis. Therefore, the AIDS may be treated as one of the organic psychosis.

AIDS IN INDIA

The dreaded disease i.e. AIDS had its origin somewhere and not in India. The United States was the first country in the world witnessed the drastic consequences of the AIDS. When they were astonished on the statistics of the number of cases of syphilis as two million in America in the year 1970, and when they were taking the preventive measures, they had suddenly experienced the violent attacks of some disease which was more dangerous than the syphilis. On knowing the dangerous effects of this disease the American Medical Association and the experts started studying what it is and wanted to find out medicines and methods of treatment. The root cause of it was traced and the virus that has caused this disease is found to be the HIV virus and the name of the disease is the AIDS. In a very short time this disease is known to the world. It rapidly spread out to several countries and India is one among them.

Experts state that AIDS is highly contagious, infectious and violent. Since it is a sex disease, it is sexually transmitted. In India the high risk groups are highly debaucherous and who show utter indifference to moral principles and behaviour. They are easily infected with this disease. The transport drivers carry goods to long distant places at inter-state level and they get contact with women who are commercial sex workers. They are the store house of all kinds of sex diseases including the AIDS. It is found that the inter-state contact is more rapid between Maharashtra and Tamil Nadu. These are the two States identified as AIDS infected States in India. The AIDS cases in other States also are considerably increasing.

Apart from the high risky groups, the groups like the less risky groups and the sophisticated groups are also getting into the drap of the AIDS. The AIDS causing atmosphere is fastly developing in India. Although the consequences of syphilis and the AIDS are almost the same the mass media of communication and the AIDS awareness organizations have created an alarming picture of the AIDS. As a result of it persons who are infected with AIDS have developed a sense of extreme fear and the feeling of helplessness. Persons of the present younger generation in India are becoming highly promiscuous in sexual liaison irrespective of age and status. Luxury and sex are becoming the fashion of the day. The present day motion picture and the Television themes have changed thoroughly the moral atmosphere of the youth. The drastic obscene scenes in motion pictures are highly stimulating the young and old of both sexes for premarital permissive promiscuous sexual activities of any type with multiple partners become the cause of some kind of venereal disease in them, ultimately ending in the some kind of venereal disease in them, ultimately ending in the infection of the HIV virus and the AIDS. The HIV virus infected cases of men and women are increasing in hospitals everyday.

Researches and experiments on AIDS are going on continuously and hopeful results are brought out. One valuable result received by the National Aids Control Society Project is that there are hopes for the children of HIV infected women. According to the AIDS Control Society Project, it is important to save the child from HIV infection. In preventing the mother-to-child transmission there is some hope yet for the already born children and to be born children of HIV infected women. The Superintendent of Kasturba Gandhi Government Hospital, Chennai (2002) said that in the year 2000 January there were many cases of HIV infected and there were about 19,000 persons attended the counselling, 14,500 were screened and 47 were treated with positive HIV and 21 persons were treated with AZI medicine and the compliances were good in all cases.

There were 25 babies born, 14 babies did not show any symptoms of HIV infection, but it was detected in three babies. However, after two months treatment the number of HIV infection was found to be one. All the screened patients were subjected to periodic check-ups upto five to fifteen years. The counselling on AIDS is an important aspect in dealing with the AIDS. Three hospitals in Chennai, Kasturba Gandhi Hospital, Ramaswamy Mudaliar Hospital, Royapuram and the Institute of Obstetrics and Gynaecology, Egmore are vigorously working on it.

It is reported by Bhattacharya (2002) that increasing number of AIDS patients are going to the Government Hospital of Thoracic Medicine, Tambaram. This is causing great concern to the authorities and to the State Government and it is becoming a tough time to organizations working on AIDS control and prevention to provide the patients adequate care. It is estimated that at least fifty fresh cases on an average are reported in the previous year (2001). This incident forces the authorities to construct additional wards to accommodate them. Out of 31 wards in the Hospital (which includes tuberculosis and cancer wards) there are four male wards, two female wards and one children ward for the AIDS. These wards here that Tamil Nadu is one of the AIDS identified States in India and it is having more number of AIDS infected patients than other states.

Since the AIDS cases are increasing everyday in Tambaram hospital, the authorities are not able to provide beds for them. The AIDS patients are put on the floor and between beds. On 2.3.2002 alone there were 234 AIDS patients undergoing treatment in various wards. The disease has reached the alarming stage in Tamil Nadu. The increase in number of the patients is the result of the intensive awareness drive. There are also equal number of tuberculosis patients getting admission in this Hospital. The AIDS patients and the tuberculosis patients are put up together in the Hospital, side by side and given treatment. It is believed that the tuberculosis is an offshoot of AIDS. The treatment is also somewhat similar to both the diseases in the beginning for reducing the intensity of infection as both are infectious diseases. In the State of Maharashtra also it is said that almost the same condition is prevailing.

POISONOUS CHEMICAL SUBSTANCE : THE ANTHRAX

Anthrax

Anthrax is a highly infectious disease of animals, especially of the cattle and the sheep, characterized by fever, enlarged spleen and swelling of throat. The plural form of this disease is *Anthraces*. It is caused by the bacterium: *Bacillus Anthracis'* (Collins, 1979). This can be transmitted to human beings and it may cause *pustule* which is a pus filled pimple or blister or both. The anthrax is a poisonous substance and it can be made more powerful poisonous material. The anthrax is produced in powder form. It is also mixed in food and water.

On knowing the danger that the anthrax bacterium can cause death to human beings, some of the terrorist organizations started manufacturing the anthrax. Afghanistan, Iraq and some of the West Asian countries manufacture the anthrax in such a way that it should kill the human beings instantly on smelling it even at a very small kill the human beings instantly on smelling it even at a very small level. The anthrax first gets into the human body through nose, ear and throat, reaches the lungs and damages the blood purification process and gets into the blood. The blood oxygenation process of the lungs is impaired.

There are two tubular systems such as *pulmonary arteries* and the *pulmonary veins* which function between heart and lungs. There are two arteries which are tubular, thick walled muscular vessels.

The pulmonary veins are tubular vessels that convey oxygen rich blood from the lungs to the heart. The oxygen depleted blood, which is channelized in bulk by the heart from various parts of the body to the lungs through the pulmonary artery for purification. The lungs purify or oxygenate the oxygen deficient blood and convey oxygen rich blood to the heart through pulmonary veins. From heart this oxygenated blood is sent through arteries to various parts of the body including the brain.

The anthrax gets into the course of blood circulation from lungs and goes to the heart and from there to the brain and destroys the brain tissues, causing behaviour disorders and finally kills the man. This is how the powerful anthrax bacterium, '*Bacillus Anthracis*' is functioning.

Anthrax damaging bodily parts and causes behaviour disorders. Some of the symptoms that appear are quite similar to other organic diseases. But certain specific symptoms are not yet correctly diagnosed. It kills man within a short period. Therefore, anthrax may be classified as one of the organic disorders.

A recent development of the terrorist network is that a series of Al-Qaeda videotapes throw some new light on Osama Bin Laden's terrorism network, which revealed some chemical gas experiments on animals. The terrorists were given lessons on making explosives. The terrorist training tactics were previously unseen images of the international terrorist mastermind and his groups. The lesson tapes obtained from inside Afghanistan show the agonizing death of the three dogs exposed to chemical agents. The experiment was conducted before the terrorist attack on United States on September 11, 2001.

The chemicals were shown to many experts including Gunaratna an expert on Al-Qaeda. He is the author of 'Inside Al-Qaeda". Gunaratna interviewed all the members of the terrorists network. He could not get the correct information. He is supposed to know everything that is going on in Al-Qaeda Camp. With all that Osama Bin Laden had maintained some secret documents of the chemicals which were not shown to Gunaratna.

Osama Bin Laden is considered to be the chief architect of the International Terrorist Movement, who was mainly responsible to attack the United States and demolish the important Trade Towers and the Pentagon. Following his terrorist tactics some other West Asian countries are also manufacturing the chemical poisonous weapons for killing their enemies. The poisonous gases and chemical materials are more powerful and can kill living organisms including human beings instantly on smelling them. It appears that these anthrax weapons are somewhat improved models of the earlier anthrax weapons.

With regard to the treatment of this disease, precautions measures should be taken in advance. But suitable medicines and methods of treatment are yet to be discovered by the medical and chemical scientists. The existing medicines and methods of treatment that are applied to animals in India and elsewhere cannot be successfully applied to human beings.

The anthrax is mostly manufactured in the form of powder to make it easy for sending it by post. It is understood that this poisonous material was sent to some well known persons by post in some of the countries. So far there is no such incidents in India. But, since the dangerous consequences are known to people in India through press and television, there is every reason for people getting panic. Therefore, the Ministry of Communication, Department of Posts, Government of India have issued a notification in the interest of public in October 20th, 2002 asking the people, under the heading of 'Anthrax–No Reason to Panic' in the Press (19.10.2001, *The Hindu*). The contents of the notification indicate that there is every chance that some persons in India may receive the anthrax by post.

The notification states, that in the context of Anthrax threat precautionary steps to identify, postal articles suspected to contain such harmful chemicals. The department is taking this opportunity made many suggestions to customers, the general public for their information, understanding and identification of such articles received in mail.

According to their suggestions, letters containing powdery or stiff material, letter containing lumpy material giving foul odour, letters, or parcels having excessive postage and addressed to well known persons, letters containing marking like 'do not open', 'to be opened by the addressee only' suspicious of unknown substance leaking from postal item, excessively taped articles, unusual smell, personal notations or greetings outside the envelope and unusual return name and address in any such suspicious letter or parcel should be immediately handed over to the police. They should wash their hands in case of such suspicious article is handled. The notification also stated that so far there has not been a single case in India of a postal article having been found to contain Anthrax. Therefore, there is no reason to panic. All these indicate that the Anthrax is a dangerous chemical substance and people should get rid of it by all means.

3

Pre- and Post-Psyche of the AIDS Patients

Some Behavioural Observations

SHEETLA PRASAD*

INTRODUCTION

Human beings are always trying to improve their living standard. A high living standard is often confused with loose morals and harmful habits. Carnal pleasure becomes the sole aim of life. This may lead to certain harmful and dangerous effects, such as the AIDS, the product of both of the situations. This newest disease which was diagnosed not more than 15 years ago, has become a challenge of the medical sciences. Researches of the AIDS are two: 1. Defective blood transfusion and the faulty sexual pleasure. The rate of AIDS development is very high by sexual abuse. About 84 per cent of the cases were reported with the effect of sex victim and only 16 per cent of the cases were reported as cause of the blood transfusion and mother to child. AIDS (Acquired Immune Deficiency Syndrome) was first time diagnosed by the young immunologist Michael Gottlieb (1981) and his research was supported by Metaigner (1983). After some early confusion the name of this disease was given a scientific name HIV

* Senior Lecturer in Psychology, Ewing Christian College, Allahabad-211 003.

(Human Immunodeficiency Virus). Immune is the human body's defence system. The deficiency in the immune system of the patient becomes weak. The perceived symptoms come after about five years. In that period the system becomes very much deficient and with high positive HIV and treatment become very difficult. Due to late processing in coming symptoms the word, 'acquired' is imposed with this name. Now some findings show that it is also a chromosomal disease and infectious parents transmit the disease to their babies. The results reveal that this disease is caused more by sexual infection than by any other cause. If majority of the cases are due to sexual union then it is in the hands of men-women to control this.

The main objective of this article is to highlight the psychological perspective of the victimized person before and after the diagnosis of AIDS.

PSYCHOLOGICAL CONDITIONS BEFORE THE DIAGNOSIS OF AIDS

Psychological conditions of the AIDS patient before the diagnosis may be ascertained with the help of detailed case histories. Normally, pleasure seeking behaviours are found in such histories. For this gain of sex pleasure, he or she does not think about what he or she is doing. This is mostly dependent upon the attitude towards sexual behaviour, information about sexual models and availability of the sex partner.

Faulty Sexual Exercise

Faulty sexual exercises are the main causes of the AIDS. The faulty sexual exercises are of five forms such as (i) Co-marital sex swinging, (ii) Sexual Sadism, (iii) Sexual Masochism, and (iv) Pedophilia, and (V) Homosexuality.

Co-marital Sex Swinging

Co-marital sex is a type of extramarital sex. Now-a-days this has become a status symbol of some elite groups. In this type of the sexual exercise wives and husbands participate openly and jointly in extramarital encounter. Extramarital means something more than what is usual, or expected, especially of sexual relations, occurring outside of marriage. An activity in addition to what has been performed usually. In some metropolitan cities the change-wife phenomena is generally occurring. Hunt (1970) reported that 2 per cent of his sample involved in swinging among them, the women proportion was high. Gilmartin (1975) assessed the psychology of this type of partners and reported that affluent and well educated people of his sample have major motive to novelty in sexual practices. Therefore, co-marital sex swinging means to be ultra-fashionable specially in seeking sexual pleasure, operating with full vigour. The persons who are engaged in this type of sexual pleasure are called swingers. Another researcher like Bartell (1970) reported that many swingers preserve marital stability through a strict prohibition against becoming emotionally involved with their swinging partners. In this situation the swinger does not care what will be in future. Their orientations are only on the sexual satisfaction with a novel stimulant.

Sexual Sadism

Sexual sadism is the major role player of the AIDS. About 10-13 per cent reported AIDS cases were due to sadism or masochism. In sexual sadism an individual attains sexual gratification through inflicting pain on sex partners. Sadism may be expressed through physical acts such as whipping, slapping or biting or verbally through teasing and sarcasm. The Freudian point of view is that sadism may allow men to exercise power over the partner and thus unconsciously resuming that they are maintaining their sex organs as with exhibition and voyeurism. Freudians suggest that such type of people suffered with castration anxiety. Sometimes this sexual sadism becomes very high. In such cases the female is affected by injury, and if this injurious part is sex organ, but not easily perceived, then the AIDS virus is developed very smoothly.

Sexual Masochism

Sexual masochism is different from sexual sadism. In sexual masochism, an individual receives sexual gratification through receiving pain from sex partners. Masochists seek not only physical punishment, but also verbal assaults for being naughty. Masochist as sadist believe that sex is dirty, and it may be that the punishment they seek permits them to cope with their guilt. Hunt (1974) found almost twice as many women as men to have received masochist pleasure and the incidences were five times as high among single as married women. Philiprice (1979) reported dyspareunia is the basic result of this type of abnormality in sexual relations. Tension, fear and anxiety are the basic prior conditions for this type of acting.

Pedophilia

This is a type of sexual abnormality in the present times and this is generally reported in newspapers often that it is practised in many places. In this abnormal sexuality state, an adult desires and engages in sexual activity with a child, who is not fit for sexual union. The child preferred by the pedophilic may be mainly the opposite sex and also may be of the same sex. Psychological findings indicate that pedophilia may occur more often in individuals who find problems in adult sexual relationships. The average age of the pedophilics was found to be around 40 years (Carson *et al.*, 1988). There are also cases of women pedophilia, playing dominant roles.

The problems and difficulties the male individuals meet with are in coping up the marital relationship with their wives. The pedophilia males show masculine inadequacy in heterosexual and homosexual activities with adults. It is because of this they are engaged in this type of activities and they are more comfortable with children, but they do not have real affection for them. Since there is physical acceptability of such children who are not appropriate for sexual activity, there are chances for the AIDS to generate easily. There are reports in newspapers recently that child sexual abuses are increasing rapidly in India, England and in some other countries.

All these four sexual abnormalities are the sexual activities, generally take place with the opposite sex. All these sexual activities may take place due to dissatisfaction and frustration caused in the sexual activity with the opposite sex.

Though homosexuality is classified as one of the sexual abnormalities, it is prevalent in the western society and it seems that it is receiving the constitutional sanction. It has been observed that homosexuality is one of the contributing phenomenon of the AIDS.

Homosexuality

Homosexuality now-a-days has taken the form of trans-sexuality. In India four cases are reported of trans-sexuality. Homosexual origin is a very controversial issue, but the person may desire for such function. This has some theoretical background. These theorists trace some prior conditions in these persons. The behavioural theorist is of the view that homosexual is reinforced by the heterosexual satisfaction. If any unexpected fear is aroused in the mind, the satisfaction in the reinforcement is reduced. For the tension reduction and gaining maximum sexual satisfaction they were attracted by the homosexuality. The psycho-analytic view is that homosexuals resolve their Oedipal and Electra Complexes in a fashion different from the majority, in the case of males (Siegelman, 1974; Ibrahim, 1976).

Immune Responses and Psychological Phenomena

Earlier researches regarding AIDS did not accept any role of psycho-social factors. But the development of new field in the area of psychology, like Psycho-Neuro-Immunology, focussed the major influence of the psychological effects on AIDS. Immune functions find, depression, psycho-social stressers and mental status (Carson, Butcher & Coleman 1988). The AIDS researches bring out the basic causes of it. There are two causes, reported for AIDS, the blood transfusion and the sexually transmitted virus. In both of the cases the immune deficiency is found in male or female or even in both. The biological cause of immune deficiency is the white blood cells. Researchers like Schleifer, Keller & Steim (1985) reported that these blood cells may be depressed with the sleep deprivation, marathon running, space flight, death of spouse and psychological depression. Jemmott & Locke (1984) reported that there is impairing effect in the immune system by mental status. According to this finding hypothalamus-pituitary-adreno-cortical (HPA) axis are responsible for the immune functioning. With the stress functioning the steroids (Adreno Cortical hormones) secrete in excessive levels. This excessive secretion impairs the immune system very gradually, but in the longer run the syndrome show in the form of AIDS.

Later AIDS researches do not positively favour the stresser (but not ignored), and the AIDS development. Researches indicated that cerebral syphilis is the major role player of AIDS, (Gabel *et al.*, 1986). Researches on this pathway indicated that severe AIDS affected patients have psychological problems like delirium, dementia, hallucination, delusion, anxiety and organic personality syndrome (Carson *et al.*, 1988). Medical sciences have approachable result in the case of AIDS captured by preventing the cerebral syphilis. In California 34 cases out of 310 were checked for preventing the cerebral syphilis.

POST- PSYCHE OF AIDS PATIENTS

AIDS patients have poor prognosis by their psychological effects. The major symptom of the AIDS patient is the cyclothymia. DSM-III-R categorized the different states in AIDS patients' psychological standard under three major categories on the basis of their severity level as cyclothymia, dysthymia 'hemia and adjustment disorder with depressed mood.

At the early stage of the AIDS, diagnosed patients suffered by cyclical mood alternation and depression. These symptoms known as cyclothymia (DSM-III-R). Studies like those Klein, Depue & Slater (1985-1986) focussed that these patients suffered with less pleasure in usual activities, low energy level, feeling of inadequacy, decreased efficiency, productivity, talkativeness and cognitive sharpness, relative disinterest in sex, pessimistic, brooding attitude. Over the time past the uncurable AIDS patients come under the category of dysthymia. In this stage all the abnormalities which were in first phase were found to exist, but some included newly which in the effect of the general depression due to bad thinking of the social environment. In this stage the patient avoids to meet his/her friends, relatives and even neighbours to a maximum level. Desire for isolation is found common in the patients. The extreme severe phase is loaded with adjustment disorder with depressed mood. Reactions of these patients are generally stressful. In this phase the diagnosis as well as prognosis become very difficult, because patients suffered with neurotic defence. They show the behaviours like chronically overactive, dominating. counter dependent, deficient in self-criticism and optimistic on their plans and schemes.

The general reactions found in all AIDS patients (after acknowledging the AIDS) are the hesitation in accepting the sharing guilt feeling hiding, avoiding medical help, seeking isolation from the society and postponing the treatment which results in worsening the state of the disease (Fig. 3.1).

AIDS IN INDIA AND THE EFFORTS OF THE GOVERNMENT

According to report of Kumudini Marathe (TOI, August 6, 1995) 40 lakhs of people have HIV positive and 2 lakhs are diagnosed as AIDS patients. Of these about 84 per cent are sexually transmitted, 10 per cent through blood transfusion and 5 per cent from mother to child. Approximately 15,000 HIV positives live in Bombay. 1041 cases on record in Maharashtra. The Government is very serious on this infectious disease. The first hospital and rehabilitation centre for the AIDS patients was set up at Gadab in the Raighad district of Maharashtra. The Indian Health Organisation (IHO), a voluntary organisation involved in checking the spread of AIDS since 1985. But unfortunately the psychological aids are not given for these effected persons though they have a lot of problems and are ready for counselling. The family of these diagnosed patients are also looking forward for the psychological aids very curiously.

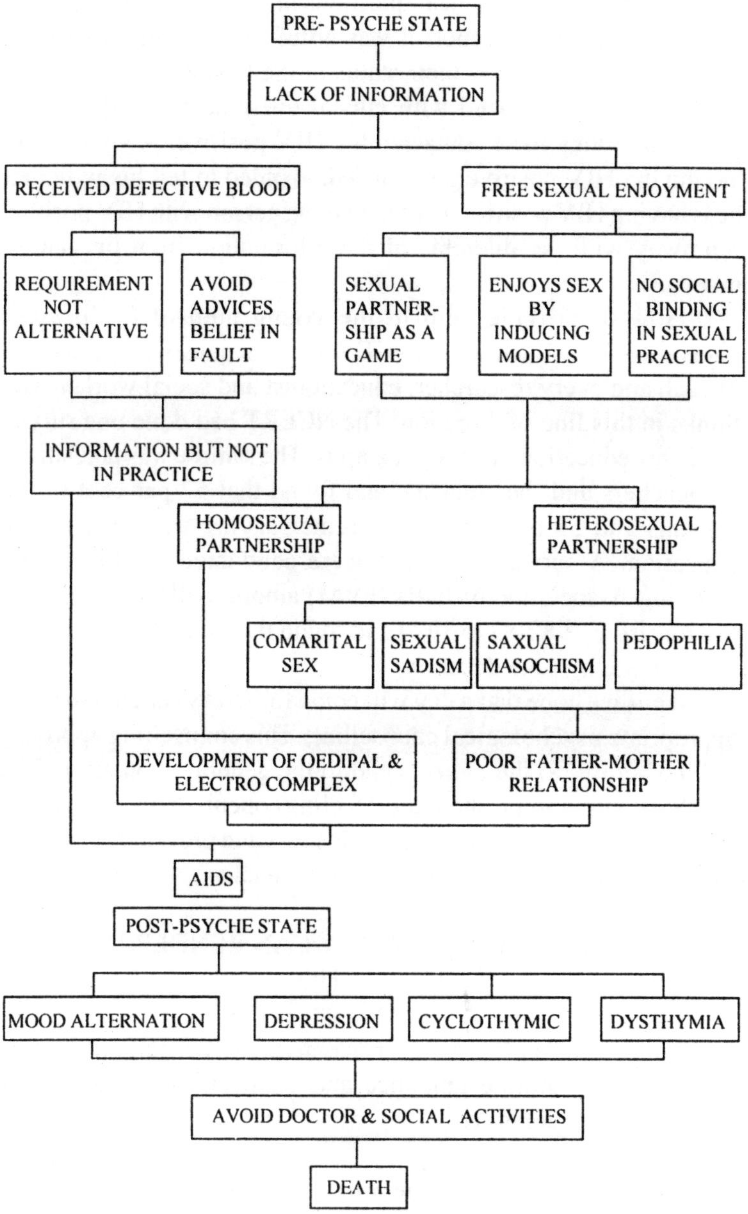

Fig. 3.1 : Diagramatic Illustration of Pre- and Post- Psyche of the AIDS Patients

Some burning psychological questions are raised by the report of Rupa Chimai. In her report it was noted that the AIDS patients have avoided to declare their status in the hospital environment. Some couples are faced with ethical dilemma when they have known that they have contacted the HIV positive. A young man having the HIV positive got married, avoided to tell his wife that he is having HIV positive. Another young person with HIV positive run away with the dilemma of the information from his family member.

How to provide help to the young men of the present generation for preventing the AIDS. It is the question in the mind of each and every researcher, educationist and social worker who thinks in this line of direction. The NCERT had done one survey about sex education in college campus. The sample was taken from the teachers and the students; and found that 57 per cent of the students and 53 per cent of the principals are in favour of sex education. A series of surveys were conducted by the Family Planning Association of India (FPAI) among college students in Madras from 1982-83 to 1994 and found that sexual activities did not increase by sex education.

Thus we hope that a day will come for AIDS patients for their appropriate psychological counselling. This counselling approach will be helpful to the patients and to the general population. The AIDS patients should share their feelings openly with the medical aid providers and should reduce their stress and prevent the cerebral syphilis in defence of the immune deficiencies.

THE SERVICES PSYCHOLOGY CAN RENDER IN AIDS PREVENTION

Psychologists can offer their services to the AIDS patients by way of providing suitable guidance and counselling. Some of the counselling methods are:

1. Creating awareness in the minds of the blood donors and the blood receivers.
2. Making of the importance in the use of disposable needles for injections.

3. Providing appropriate sex education for the adolescent students and young adults.
4. Using pornographic material in the teaching to reduce the curiosity of the body organs among the adolescents and young adults.
5. Providing satisfactory answer about sex functions and about psychological health to the concerned individuals.
6. Explaining about the consequences of their abnormal functioning of sexual behaviour and making them to know how harmful the future is going to be for the adolescents and young adults.
7. Educational training for the adjustment with the opposite sex related behaviour.
8. Teaching moral principles and disseminating right knowledge in sex related behaviour.

4

AIDS Awareness and Prevention

R.S. MANI*

INTRODUCTION

Human immunity against foreign bodies and diseases are maintained by (i) Leucocytes-white blood corpuscles, (ii) T-cells, white blood corpuscles engulf the foreign particle and destroy it. When the need arises WBC multiply in the required number to solve the problem. At the molecular level, T-cell effector and regular functions are mediated by secreted lymphokines and monokines, e.g. by interferons, interlinking, migration inhibitory factors, lymphotoxins etc. These soluble substances are the intracelluar messengers that regulate interaction between monocytes, T and B lymphocytes and are involved in homeostatic regulation and expression of immunity and inflammation (Sadhukhan, *et al.*, 1993). The T-cells (T-lymphocytes) produce antibody and these antibodies are able to destroy the foreign organisms or substances. Human Immuno Virus (HIV) is responsible for causing Acquired Immune Deficiency Syndrome (AIDS).

* Reader in Education (CASE), Faculty of Education and Psychology, M.S. University of Baroda, Vadodara-390 002.

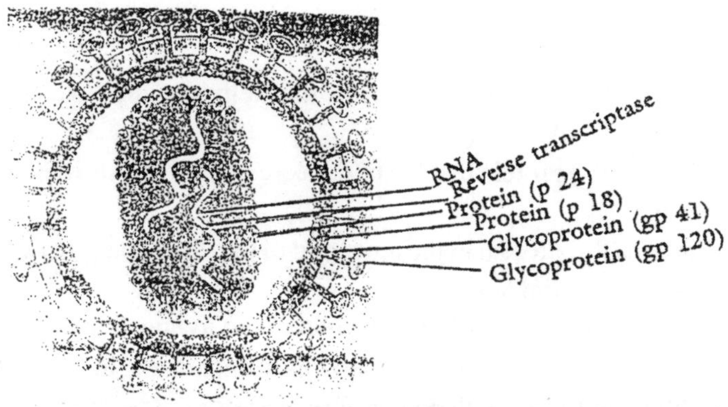

Figure 4.1 : Model of HIV
Source: Banergia 1992, pp. 5

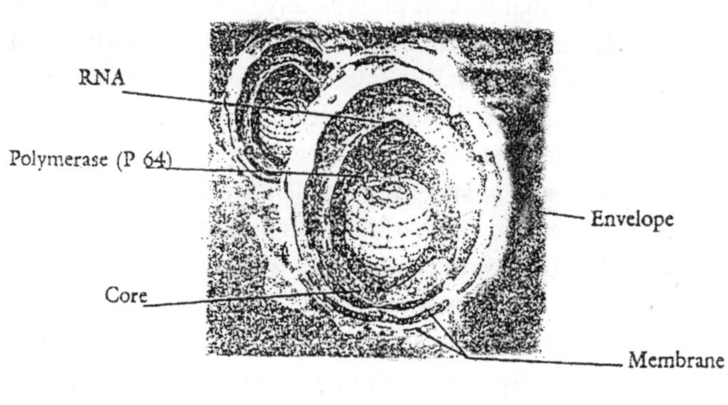

AIDS Virus (HIV) : How it looks
Figure 4.2: AIDS VIRUS : The Inner View
Source: Banergia, 1992, pp. 9

STRUCTURE OF HUMAN IMMUNE DEFICIENCY SYNDROME

1. RNA : Ribonucleic Acid
   The genetic material.
2. Reverse transcriptase the enzyme that helps the virus to convert RNA to DNA.
3. Protein (P_{24}) protein that forms the core of the virus surrounding RNA.
4. Protein (P_{18}) protein in the inner part of the virus that is believed to produce viral surface.
5. Glyco-protein (gP_{41}) helps the outer coat to attack the cells.
6. Glyco-protein (gP_{120}) helps the virus to anchor and get attached to the cell to attack them.
7. Fat layer–the outer coat of the virus.

HIV, generally, enters through blood and gets attached to a molecule called CD_4 which is present on the surface of the T-cells. Protein on the exterior envelope of the virus bind to the CD_4 molecule and the membranes of the virus and the T-cell fuse. As a result, RNA, proteins and enzymes of HIV enter the T-cell. It is interesting to note that HIV binds with any other white blood cells containing CD_4 and can remain dormant for few months (3 to 6 months) to many years. At this stage, it is difficult to identify the HIV through blood test. The RNA, protein and enzymes of HIV after entering cytoplasm of T-cell, and enzyme called 'reverse transcriptase' present in HIV converts RNA into DNA.

The newly formed DNA of HIV enters the nucleus of T-cell. When T-cell multiplies, the virus DNA is also copied. A person infected with HIV may contain billions of cells containing the HIV DNA. The T-cell containing HIV DNA cannot produce new viruses unless the RNA is able to make its own copies. The infected T-cell produces enzymes for multiplication of new viruses, with the help of messenger RNA transcription takes place. The m-RNA of HIV is released into the cytoplasm. In cytoplasm, the HIV uses T-cell's protein making mechanism to make long chains of proteins and enzymes of HIV. The m-RNA acts as a template for production of

HIV proteins and enzymes. The T_4 lymphocyte is destroyed. The T_4 lymphocyte (of the infected T-cell) cannot induce other immune cells called B lymphocytes to produce disease fighting antibodies; it also fails to recognize the foreign substances or antigens and fail to proliferate.

The newly made HIV proteins, enzymes and RNA collect inside the wall of the infected T-cell. At the same time, the proteins that form the outer layer of the virus collect within the wall of the infected T-cell. An immature particle of the virus is formed and separates from the infected T-cell. This immature virus cannot spread the infection to other people. The long chains of proteins and enzymes formed inside the infected cell are cut into smaller pieces by a specific enzyme of the virus called protease. This step results in formation of viral particles that can spread infection to other T-cells. Finally, lose their ability to produce interleukin-2 (Il-2), a molecule that enhances the growth of T-cells and helps to stimulate their response to foreign antigens.

It is necessary to know that AIDS may remain dormant for years after infection. Usually it takes even 10 years before a person with HIV infection shows full signs or symptoms of the illness. AIDS does not kill by itself but by breaking down the body's natural biological immune system it allows ordinary diseases like, diarrhoea, fever, pneumonia, tuberculosis, cancer, etc. to manifest and kill the patient with impunity (Banerjea, 1992).

HIV can only be infected by blood to blood transmission and it is not at all contagious as the virus does not survive more than 10 minutes outside the body. The virus does not survive when the blood is dried up or it does not have a carrier. Pushpa Khurana (1989) states that green monkeys in Africa were infected by HIV and these monkeys blood through biting Africans have got HIV. However, it is well established through various studies that HIV is transmitted only through blood to blood contact for considerable period to cause infection.

HISTORY OF AIDS

Rajamanickam, (1992) in a research study states that Ho and his associates (1985) were the first to isolate and identify the HIV from the cerebrospinal fluid and neural tissues. Ho's patients have demonstrated certain neurological symptoms. These symptoms were quite similar to the symptoms exhibited by Nurnberg's patients which had the characteristics of what is known as AIDS dementia complex (ADC). This was the first evidence to conclude and to show that the HIV is capable of crossing the brain-blood barrier which is considered to be the defence mechanism. This defence mechanism normally permits only oxygen, nutrients and waste to pass through between the blood vessels and the cerebrospinal fluid. If the HIV gets access directly to the brain to cause ADC, it is very strange. The HIV somehow is able to contact the brain and becomes responsible for the cause of ADC.

AIDS is a sexually transmitted disease. There are several cases of homosexuals suffering from AIDS in USA. The tissue in the anus allows easy mixing of infected blood with the normal person. The sexual partners generally have more chances of contacting AIDS. The initial AIDS cases reported in India were from the sexual partners in Chennai and Mumbai. In India, the National AIDS campaign has provided to sexual partners with condoms for protecting against AIDS. AIDS are reported with narcotics and regular drug abusers.

Banerjea, (1992) reports that HIV was first recognized in 1983 in the Pasteur Institute in Paris and then in 1985 in the National Cancer Institute in Bethesda, USA, of the HIV (Human Immuno Deficiency Virus) which is believed to cause the dreadful disease AIDS (Acquired Immuno Deficiency Syndrome). Kowlas (2002) has recently developed a data base on HIV/AIDS in Subsaharan Africa region.

HOW AIDS SPREAD

HIV infection spreads through generally five ways:

1. Sexual intercourse (homeosexual or heterosexual) with the infected person.
2. Blood transfusion.
3. Infections (when syringe and needles are not disposed).

4. When infected blood contacts any cut in the skin or injury.
5. Mother-to-child transmission during pregnancy (for HIV passes through placenta to the child) or delivery. HIV is very small in size and it can pass through very fine filter paper or membrane.

Rate of Spread of AIDS

Banerjea, (1992) states that in USA the number of paediatric AIDS cases rose four-fold between 1985 and 1990, and in Europe the increase has been five-fold during the same period. AIDS has spread worldwide. 'An estimated 23 million people worldwide are reported to be living with HIV infection. All of them will develop AIDS within the next ten years. About eighty thousand people worldwide are estimated to be infected with HIV infection per day' (*Health Update*, 1999). Ninety per cent of people with HIV infections are in developing world and of these the majority are in sub-saharan Africa. According to the estimates of the World Health Organisation, about thirty to forty million people all over the world will be infected by HIV by the year 2002 and of these eight to ten million people will develop AIDS, Kenya and Zambia have regular and thorough screening of blood samples for testing AIDS before going for blood transfusion.

Health Update (1999) reports that the first AIDS case in India was reported in 1986 from Madras (Chennai). In the past one and half decades HIV infection has rapidly spread all over the country. By March 1998, the National AIDS Control Organization had reported that a total of seventy-one thousand, four hundred people were having HIV infection from among 3.2 million people who were tested for it.

During the same period, a total of five thousand one hundred forty five people had been reported to have developed AIDS of these, about eighty per cent were males and twenty per cent females. Almost eighty nine per cent people with AIDS were in the age group of fifteen to forty-four years, which are the most economically productive years for any individual. Maharashtra State has reported the maximum number of HIV infections followed by Tamil Nadu and Manipur (*Health Update*, 1999).

How to Test HIV Infection ?

There are two well accepted tests to find the infection of HIV.

1. *Elisa Test*: In this test HIV antibodies are detected. This test is repeated (3 times) in order to confirm the infection. On positive testing for HIV, the individual needs to go for another test namely Western Blot Test.
2. *Western Blot Test detects antibodies to HIV*: A western blot test is said to be positive if the test shows reactivity to the antigens of at least two of the following components of HIV P-24, GP-41 and GP-160. A negative test is one which does not indicate antibodies to any of the above components of the virus. In case there is reactivity to one or more antigens only, or if there is weak reaction, the test result is said to be doubtful.
3. *Test to detect HIV Polymerase Chain Reaction (PCR) Test*: These tests can indicate the presence of the virus in new born babies or adults within a week of their getting HIV infection. The PCR tests can also estimate the number of viruses in the blood and therefore, the PCR test is used to assess the progress of the disease (Source *Health Update*, 1999).
4. *Test to estimate the number of T cells in the blood*: Estimating the number of T cells in the blood or the total CD_4 count in the blood is used for identifying the stage of HIV infection, plan the most suited treatment option and diagnose AIDS. It can also be used to decide whether specific preventive measures are desirable for opportunistic infections or not. The decline in CD_4 cells (T cells) indicates increased risk of getting infections.

SYMPTOMS OF AIDS

AIDS may not show up any symptom for ten years. However, there are certain major signs to infer AIDS. They are :

1. Diarrhoea associated with excessive loss of weight.

2. Chronic cough (Cough may be due to other reasons).
3. Enlarged lymph nodes (such as armpits, neck and groin), for other reasons also lymph nodes enlarge.
4. Chronic fever lasting for a month.
5. Pneumonia
6. Tuberculosis
7. Cancer (Kaposi's Sarcoma) skin cancer.

Preventive Measures against AIDS

1. Avoiding multiple sex partners.
2. Using fresh syringe and needle or dispensing syringe and needle in injections.
3. Demand in the saloon for the use of a fresh blade.
4. Ask for AIDS test before transfusion of blood.
5. Never recycle the blood stained bandage, cloth, needle or syringe.
6. Breast milk is the best food and allow your child to be breast fed.
7. Some physician's suggest that even a mother with AIDS disease need to feed her baby with breast milk.
8. Milk banks established in Hospitals need to test for AIDS and provide milk to the children.
9. The blood banks need to regularly check for AIDS when the blood is donated and again test before giving blood transfusion. The government needs to strictly regulate this protocol and frame appropriate laws. Countries such as Kenya and Zambia are already ahead of us in strict monitoring of blood testing for AIDS in blood banks.
10. AIDS patients need to be strictly monitored for preventing further infection. They need to be looked at sympathetically and their needs must be met urgently.
11. Narcotics and drug addicts need to be monitored for a longer period in order to check for AIDS.
12. Regular sexual partners need to be monitored for a longer period by the government and they need to be provided condoms free of cost.

13. Mexico has introduced a special chapter on AIDS in the Biology text books used in their schools and have a round-the-clock counselling hot-line service. In India, also there is a need to introduce a special chapter on AIDS in Biology text books in schools and provide for a round-the-clock counselling hot-line service.
14. Video-films on AIDS and modes of preventive measures need to be shown to all students.
15. Film theatres must show documentary on AIDS before screening any movie.
16. The internet sites on AIDS and preventive measures need to be made more popular for the cybernet users.
17. Radio bulletins must be broadcasted periodically on AIDS and its prevention.
18. The literature on AIDS and its prevention must be made available to everyone at low cost in all Indian languages. Government must subsidise the production of AIDS educational material and publications.
19. The local folklore, skits, plays, dramas on AIDS prevention messages will educate the illiterate public.
20. Government must produce condoms in great number and popularise its use.
21. Billboards can be prepared in local languages about AIDS and its prevention and be displayed in public places prominently for educating the public.
22. P.H.Cs. in rural areas and paramedics need to be educated to identify AIDS cases if any and refer them to hospitals for treatment and promote preventive measures.
23. The research concerning immunological aspects need to be strengthened in order to understand the nature of the virus and find suitable medicine within the country or abroad.
24. Elisa and Western Blot Test are costly. The Government of India through the National AIDS surveillance programme in 43 centres need to develop and strengthen testing facility at reasonably low cost.

25. Illiteracy, poverty and malnutrition are prevalent in many States. These factors increase the chances for the development of the AIDS. The efforts need to be made to increase the general standard of living.

5

AIDS Dementia and Related Diseases in India and in Other Countries

M. RAJAMANICKAM

INTRODUCTION

The development of human sciences such as psychology, psychiatry, psychopathology, psychopharmacology, neuropsychology and biological psychology, yielded vast range of information about human psycho-physical life and mental life. The information and knowledge provided by these sciences are mostly positive and some negative. Physically and mentally man has to live in the midst of perils, exposing to dangers in his living environmental conditions. As a result of it he has to struggle hard to get rid of the live inconveniences, discomforts and dangers. However, he has carefully planned his life for a continued happy living, he has to face great misfortunes and dangers from various sources. The misfortunes, dangers and circumstances not only cause inconveniences to his happy and comfortable life, but also affect him physically and mentally. He cannot escape from the physical and mental diseases of various types which not only cause his life miserable and wretched, but also make him to suffer severely and die. He cannot escape from this course of life.

The scientific and technological development and the developments in medicine and treatment techniques however advanced cent-per-cent cure and recovery from the diseases are not possible. The epidemic diseases are attacking or affecting many people simultaneously in a community or area. There will be widespread occurrences of these diseases. For example an influenza, epidemic, a highly contagious and often epidemic, a viral disease plague, a highly contagious disease with a high fatality rates the cholera, an acute infectious disease characterised by severe diarrhoea caused by ingestion of water or food contaminated with bacterium vibrio comma, yellow fever an acute infectious disease characterized by fever, haeomorrhages, vomiting of blood and jaundice caused a virus transmitted by the bite of a female mosquito of the species *Ardes Aegypti*.

CANCER

The other highly infectious disease which caused death for millions of people is cancer, a type of malignant tumour caused by abnormal and uncontrolled cell divisions, may spread through the lymphatic system or blood stream to other parts of the body including the brain and becomes a fatal. There are several causes attributed to cancer. The most common cause of cancer is using tobacco. Tobacco is used in various forms like smoking in cigarette, cigar, beedi, pipe and also tobacco is used with beetle leaves. Tobacco was brought to Europe by Columbus at the end of fifteenth century, Columbus and his sailors when first landed in West Indies, had contact with the West Indians. There was intermixture of races in various forms. Apart from the sexual contact with the West Indian women, Columbus and his sailors also adapted the cultural habits of the West Indies. One of the important habits acquired from them was the use of tobacco. But the Europeans did not want to use it in its original form. They used it in cigarettes. In a very short period the sailors and the merchants started imitating the West Indians' smoking habits using rolled leaves of tobacco and to have the experience of the West Indies. The experiences made them craving for the tobacco. If tobacco was not smoked, it was chewed and also it was made into powder and inhaled as snuff.

When the use of tobacco became very widespread all over the world, there were increasing mortality rates among the smokers or tobacco users. Researches were conducted and found that smokers and tobacco users have developed lungs cancer of larynx and of the esophagus, and also a number of cardiovascular diseases. According to the study of Jaffe (1985) the most harmful components in the smoke from the burning tobacco are nicotine, carbon monoxide and tar. These are known as *carcinogens,* the substances which produce cancer. Jaffe states that in United States persons between thirty and thirty five years, who were smokers have the mortality rate twice than that of non-smokers after developing lung cancer, which destroyed the lung tissues.

The more alarming information from Werner (1977) is that of smoking among the teenagers in United States, both boys and girls. They immitate the stars of motion picture in smoking. Once the young people started smoking, it is very difficult for them to give it up and ultimately they die of cancer. Most people accept smoking causes health hazards, but they continue to smoke which might be called as suicidal activity. The most astonishing incident is that Sigmund Freud was an addict of smoking cigar, knowing pretty well that it causes cancer. At last he had the mouth cancer and died. Bennett (1980) has observed that women who were smokers gave birth to children with lower weights and with defects. Indians both men and women in rural areas above forty years indiscriminately use tobacco chewing in various forms. Adolescent boys and young adults smoke beedies and cigarettes both in urban and rural areas. These people meet with early death not knowing the cause of it or suffer from cancer for very long period and die.

Recent researches in biological science throw some new light on cancer. One of the works was the role of psychological factors as the cause of cancer. Greer (1983) has explored the important psychological influences as the causes and outcomes of cancer. Articles often appear giving warning to the readers of newspapers and magazines about the connection between emotions and cancer. Are the emotional states promote the cause of cancer? There are studies on personality traits which atribute the likelihood of causing cancer by emotional states and stresses. Greer (1993) had conducted an experiment on this problem among the college students and found that depression and feeling of hopelessness have been associated with cancer. It was also observed that life long suppression of anger caused breast cancer in women.

Cancer Development in Older Adults

Cancer is an infectious disease which is caused by viruses, bacteria or microorganisms. Though there are medicines and methods of treatment people suffer from it and die. It is observed in some of the recent researches at Dana-Farer Cancer Institute, which has provided some new evidences for a theory of why incidences of certain cancers grow and found common in older adults. The theory is that in the tissues that are undergoing continual process, the cells die and are replaced throughout the life. This process takes place in the skin, breast in the case of women, prostate in the case of men and in colon (a part of the large intestine). This results in a genetic mutation causing some cells to divide even after their chromosomes have lost their protective protein ends, called teleomeres. As a result of this the chromosomes that fuse together in abnormal ways create chaos in the genetic programme of the cells and placing them on the path towards cancer.

The results of a very recent researches performed by Ronald De Pinho and his associates were published in the journal of *Nature* reproduced in *Medical Science* (2001). These results are involved in the development of a new strain of mice, whose ability is to develop certain cancers which resembled that of humans. Normally mice with flaws in their genetic 'brakes' against cancer develop *lymphomes* and *malignamics* known as *sarcomes* in genes and in the connective tissues. In older adults however, tumours tend to arise in epithelial cells. These cells die regularly and also are replaced. This takes place in the interior of certain organs of the body.

According to the study made by De Pinho and others in humans, the telemeres shorten each time a cell, divides until they become so short that they can no longer protect the chromosomes from damage. But at a stage the cells normally stop dividing, which is called the '*Heylick Limit*'. However, a genetic error enables them to bypass the '*hayflick limit*' and continue the process of dividing even though their chromosomes are virtually short of chromosomes. This stage is known as crisis, the cells chromosomes begin to break and fuse in abnormal places. When these chromosomes rearrangements occur, there will be very rapid gains and losses of genetic information within cells. This process is known as crisis which gives rise to pre-cancerous cells that begin to form a primary tumour. But it cannot take place until telemore function is restored. At this stage full development of the cancer has taken place. This is caused by reactivation of the *enzyme telemerase*, rebuilding and stabilizing the cells' telemeres.

We have known for long time that cancer is associated with age. De Pinho, one of the authors, remarked that we know that it tends to occur in epithelial cells in older adults and the chromosomal structure of these cancer cells is very complex.

TUBERCULOSIS

The other highly infectious disease which is caused by the micro-organisms is the tuberculosis. It is a communicable disease caused by infections with the *tubercle bacillus* most frequently affecting the lungs (pulmonary tuberculosis). It is also called *Consumption Phthisis.* Tuberculosis is mainly caused by *chronic asthma*. If the chronic asthma is not treated properly in time it results in developing to the next stage, the tuberculosis. Though tuberculosis is generally said to be caused by micro organisms like the virus, bacteria, fungi and other germs, it is also caused by the diseased brain tumour cells transferred to lungs. This is caharacterized by constant fever and headaches and the person feels weak and not in a state to carry out his normal work. It needs immediate diagnosis and suitable treatment.

DEVELOPMENT OF THE DREADED DISEASE

The mass media of communication such as the newspapers, magazines, radio and television and other publication sections of the Government, both the State and the Centre in the recent past were seriously engaged in writing and in broadcasting about one serious matter with all their efforts to draw the attention of the people of the nation. It is about the dreaded and fatal disease, the AIDS. Whether people know about it or not the publicity and propaganda machineries have caused panic among the people. People in the beginning did not know what sort of disease it is. Then gradually they began to understand what it is and what it causes.

But one important matter about this disease, AIDS is that the general public did not pay so much seriousness as to take sufficient precautionary measures. All the publicities and awareness programmes highlighted by the concerned organizations and the medical scientists were taken by the people that it was not for them. But, soon the consequences of this disease began to appear and persons who were infected with this disease were found to be suffering and were going in search of suitable medicine and methods of treatment. Persons who were infected (which is an infectious disease) with this disease and when came to know that it is the AIDS, they were very much afraid of it and also ashamed of revealing it. AIDS awareness propaganda organizations often speak of the disastrous consequences of this disease. They say that it is infectious, contagious violent, manmade and it is rooted in human sexual activities and it is incurable and has no medicine.

Though people were known all these happenings the disease is caused in large number and prevailing in India, mostly in Tamil Nadu, Andhra Pradesh and Maharashtra States. It is not caused by the environmental and water pollutions like the epidemic diseases. It is man who created it for himself to destroy himself by having sexual intercourse with a person (male or female) who is infected with a particular type of virus.

Filtering HIV Virus from the Patients' Blood

Large number of infectious cases were reported in the hospitals of United States and the cases were very serious and the ordinary methods of treatment with the existing medicines have failed to cure the disease. This was baffling the medical and biological scientists. Researches in various institutions were started to invent new medicines, equipments and methods of treatment. It was at last identified that the disease was caused by the HIV virus and the disease was acquired immune deficiency syndrome (AIDS). Scientists who were on this disease have stated that the HIV virus is unfilterable and very difficult to control it.

Several companies started to find out devices to control the HIV virus by inventing equipments that could filter and control the disease. There were also controversies on the research results published earlier.

The early researches have declared that HIV virus is infilterable from the patients' blood. But a device is found from the later development by a company in California. According to this development, a device could be used in conjunction with antivetroviral drugs, which slow down the progress of AIDS by lowering the levels of the virus. Unlike drugs, though it should have no side effects, nor should the virus be able to develop resistance. This device is called the *HIV-Hemopurifier* . This comes in a cartridge that fits into kidney dialysis machines. It contains hallow fibres with pores just large enough for the virus to pass through.

Inside the fibres there are leads coated with antibiotics that bind to GP 120 protein found on the surface of HIV as well as antisense DNA that binds to virual RNA. As in the case of normal dialysis, the intention is to pass blood through the cartridge and back into the patient. The viruses that enter the nerve fibres should attach to the beads like parts. The manufacturer of the instrument states that in preclinical trials the mechanism or the device removed 90 per cent of the HIV from the contaminated fluid part of the blood (plasma). This idea of formulating the mechanism (device) came from Jublian Ambrus of the State University of New York of Buffalo.

There were also different versions of this mechanism (device) that could be used to filter out other viruses also. The viruses are such as *hepatitis-C virus* and also heavy metals. The researches of the National Institute of Health (U.S.) state that it is a clear approach. But they make remarks of this device that the company which manufactures this instrument should prove the function on a real patient. According to them there is an important issue with the device that the GP-120 proteins are like the stalks, very weak or fragile and can be easily broken off. The resulting bald virus particles could easily pass through the filter without being captured. The role of GP-120 protein is to help the HIV enter the cells, the bald virus might be still able to do this, according to the researches there is also another problem that is, the process of dialysis is taking too much time and the equipment is very expensive. The blood dialysis treatment for kidney patients take about four hours. These problems in this device should be rectified for a successful process of filteration.

Once, if they are successful, in controlling the HIV virus either through this equipment or any other equipment it is possible to eradicate this disease just like other diseases. But the main problem with this disease is that it is rooted in human sex life which is a very sensitive area to deal with it experimentally.

The HIV Invasion Results in Melting Down of the Genes

Research findings reveal many new informations about the HIV virus and the AIDS. The research documents show that the attack of the HIV virus on the immune cells may also help to fight the infection. This was observed by the researchers who have observed the varied stages of the genetic destruction in a larger level made by the virus. This was the result of the research published by the researchers in *Nature* (2001). The malignant HIV virus infects and kills the T-cells in the blood, which normally protect against the infection. The T-cells are the lymphocytes, the immune system cells. There are two different classes of lymphocytes. They are B and T. These two are the mediate types of immunological responses. Thus the T-lymphocyte is and immune system cell that attacks any foreign microbes or tissues and kills them. Therefore, it is also called the 'kill cell'. Ultimately it wipes out the immune system and causes the AIDS. This occurs very rapidly and in ruthless manner.

The *Nature* has reported further, that Corbeil and his Co-workers (2001), after dealing with the T-cells with the virus, used the gene chips, destroyed by the virus, and regulated the activity of about seven thousand genes and they have taken about three days. This has become a worldwide survey of the process of infection. In this experimental survey it was observed that the virus rapidly shut-down the T-cell genes and more than five hundred genes died within thirty minutes. The group of the died genes were observed by the experimenters.

The HIV virus violently takes away the cell's protein-protection system for its own processes of setting up the operation of intense viral reproduction and ultimately putting the cell into death. The virus takes over the cell. The newly designed *bio-informatics software device* helped the researchers to interpret with a wealth of information. They have found that each gene on the chip was associated with important words to describe the function. It was found that there were groups of genes on the pathways that are aimed by the HIV virus. This process revealed that energy-production and the DNA-repair pathways are changed. But the cellular pathways and the cell-death genes are activated. These are the results released by an AIDS vaccine research centre in Bethesda, Maryland, U.S. (2001). These results are in contrast to the previous studies about the cells. The previous studies were focussed on the cells' response to HIV on individual gene products, but this study to some extent generalizes the effects of HIV virus (2001).

As soon as there is HIV virus infection, many T-cells are killed. The exact procedure or the method the virus performs this act has to be traced. The activation of the intrinsic cell-death genes seem to be that the cell kills itself in its attempt to stop the spread of the virus. After this dropout the T-cell strength is stablished at a level that could determine as to how long the AIDS patients are likely to survive.

HIV-AIDS in African Countries

The United Nations also are keeping watch over the consequences of the AIDS all over the world. It was observed by a senior UN official and reported that the AIDS compounds woes in Africa.

According to the UN official (2002) the AIDS epidemic in Southern Africa compounds the regional drought and hunger to create a crisis like no other that threatens more than fourteen million people. The United Nations deputy emergency relief co-ordinator, Carolyn McAskie (2002) has said that the United Nations and the regional Governments believed that the number of people affected is growing more rapidly than they expected. According to them the estimate has increased from 12.8 million to 14.4 million in a population of fifty six million. Half of the hungry people are in Zimbabwe. The Director of the U.N. World Food Programme had visited many countries in Africa and observed the situation prevailing there.

The erratic rains have inflicted drought in many areas and also the excess rains in some places, both have seriously reduced the staple crops. The drought stricken people already have serious problems in agricultural production, health care, and education. But it is the AIDS that makes this drought more serious. The regions have been hit more seriously than any other parts of the world by HIV virus, the virus that causes the AIDS.

An information released from Washington (U.S.) has provided a statistics that many countries in the world have HIV infected AIDS persons. It was a global survey made by an American organization. According to the organization, India is the country which is very much threatened with AIDS, a disease caused by indiscriminate sexual contacts. The report states that among the world nations India finds the first place in AIDS (2002). It has been estimated that in the year 2010, India will be having twenty five million AIDS patients. In India about sixty per cent of the commercial sex women workers have the AIDS. The lorry drivers who carry goods to distant places have been infected with the HIV virus, and suffer from the AIDS. It is estimated that fifteen per cent of the drivers in general have AIDS disease. The other countries which are infected with the HIV-AIDS disease, are China, Russia, Nigeria, Ethiopia, Siam and Indo-China.

A Johannesburg (2002) information states that the former South African President, Nelson Mandela has disclosed that three of his relatives have died of AIDS. Mandela, who has actively promoted AIDS awareness since stepping down from the Presidentship in 1999, said that his niece and his nephew's two sons died of AIDS in the Eastern Transkei region. It is estimated that 4.7 million South Africans, one in every nine is HIV positive infected person. The disease remains highly stigmatized among the rural communities. Mandela has stated that the Government repeatedly refused to treat the AIDS sufferers with medicine, stating that they are unaffordable and also their safety is not assured. In such a situation the AIDS patients have no other go except to die down.

Controversial Theory about the HIV's Origins

The AIDS is caused by the HIV virus which is unfilterable, and uncontrolled, highly contagious and infectious. It has baffled and mystified the medical scientists for a long time. They were struggling very seriously to bring it under control. Several researches were carried out and the results of these researches presented a controversial theory about the origin of the HIV virus.

One theory is that the AIDS pandemic was not caused by Polio Vaccines tested in Africa in the 1950s. This was the view held by several teams of researchers. But what is needed, is their research works should settle the problem once for all. The theory was questioned by several medical scientists and thus it had become a controversial theory. The theory was put forth by Edward Cooper (1991) in his book, *The River* in 1999. Cooper's claim was that tissues from chimpanzees were used to prepare the CHAT vaccine and was given to about one million people in the country of Democratic Republic of Cango. According to Cooper some batches of the vaccine became contaminated with SIV, which is the chimpanzee version of HIV, allowing the virus to jump to humans. But the Wister Institute of Philadelphia which make the vaccine, insisted that only Macaques were used. Macaques, are the any of the various old world monkeys of the genus (a type of monkeys).

This theory has been tested by two teams of researchers. One team was led by Simon Wain Holson of the Pasteur Institute in Paris and Neil Berry of Eritains National Institute of Biological Standards and Control (NIBSC) in Hertfordshire have analysed the old stocks of the vaccine. They released the results stating that there was no trace of HIV, SIV or the chimp DNA. But they have found the Macaque DNA. This result confirmed that the vaccine was prepared from Macaque cells. But Cooper did not accept it and dismissed the results presented at the meeting of the Royal Society in London in 2000, stating that the key batches of the vaccine was no longer in existence.

But Barry's team of researchers have managed to find a vital of Vaccine 10-11 at the NIBSC that originally received from Wistar Institute in 1958. Hooper specifically implicated the batch 10A-11. Thereby that this finding too was from SIV, and significantly rejected and did not support his theory. Another team headed by Edward Homes of Oxford University has created the Fullest evolutionary tree, so far from HIV by comparing the DNA of 197 strains, (the racial stock of the monkeys) from Cango. The tree suggested that the virus jumped from chimpanzee to humans years before the vaccination campaign was started (*New Scientist*).

HIV-AIDS IN CHINA

China is one of the countries identified as AIDS infected. There are organizations in China taking care of it and making intense studies and valuable results have been brought out. Chinese AIDS campaigner has expressed a disgraceful note. It was with regard to HIV tainted blood transfusions which infected hundreds of thousand of villagers. Wan Yanhai, an outspoken critic of Beijing has played as an AIDS critic. But what he has stated was not correct. Some estimates say that there are six million Chinese infected with HIV positive. A forecast stated that the figure may increase to twenty million in 2010. But the Government Authorities disagreed with this figure and stated that the number could be only six lakhs (2002).

Studies on AIDS in African countries are going on and valuable information on it are released now and then. Addis Ababa is the capital city of Ethiopia, where representatives of fourteen countries in central and eastern Africa were assembled and had discussion on the fast spreading AIDS. They have decided to have a new national action plans to tackle the HIV-AIDS and boost regional contacts. There were about one hundred delegates made commitments at national level and personality. An AIDS conference was held in Addis Ababa under the sponsorship of the U.N. Development Programme and representatives from all the countries of Central and Eastern Africa participated and resolved to fight the AIDS at all levels.

HIV-AIDS : INDIA – ANDHRA PRADESH

Organizations both Government and private pay special attention to control and eradicate the fast spreading HIV-AIDS disease by taking different type of efforts. The gravest consequences have been realized very seriously first by the Americans. Medical scientists started conducting experiments and researches, devicing equipments and methods of treatment. The Americans not only interested in controlling this disease in United States, but also all over the world. They send experts to study the situation and also provide all sorts of help to deal with this disease.

The Bill and Melinds Gates Foundation has sent a team of experts under the leadership of Bill Gates who is the chief of microsoft to supervise the on going projects in India to control the spread of HIV-AIDS during November 2002. It was said that Bill Gates was expected to declare a long range strategic commitment to support the country's efforts to solve the spread of HIV-AIDS. Gate's visit was to examine the progress of the project that has been undertaken by the Andhra Pradesh Government in collaboration with the United States (2001) AID's Programme for appropriate Technologies in Health and with the support of the Foundation to introduce Hapatitis-B Vaccine to strengthen the overall infant immunisation programme in the State. The foundation had provided with a grant of twenty million Dollars for this purpose.

There are reports of high incidence of HIV positive cases in Andhra Pradesh which cause great concern to the Government as it is becoming a very big health and social problem in the State. The cases were treated in maternity hospitals. The Government is collecting the statistics and reviewing them. The latest and urgent attention is to prevent mother-to-child transmission (PMTCT) of the HIV virus in the State that has attracted nationwide attention. This has resulted for an urgent consultation between the National AIDS Control Organization (NACO) and the AIDS control society officials (Chandrakanth, 2002). Efforts are made to study whether the cases are pertaining to the cases taken to the hospital directly or last minute referred cases for admission in the hospitals.

The AIDS control projects are working in fourteen teaching hospitals in the State, but number of average cases are only 2.3 per cent except in Vijayawada University Hospital, where there were about ten percentage of incidences. The cases reported in Visakhapatnam hospitals were found to be 1.1and 3.9 per cent. There are also reported cases in Chittoor, East Godavari, Guntur, Ananthapur, Kurnool, Warangal, Hyderabad and Secundrabad. On the whole the State average of AIDS infected cases are 2.3 per cent.

Every year there are about sixteen lakhs of delivery cases and there are about 13,000 pregnant women who are infected with HIV positive cases. The other highly prevalent States are Maharashtra, Karnataka, Tamil Nadu, Nagaland and Manipur. There are about eleven centres in six States identified for the pilot project for intensive and extensive study. A feasibility study was made at the Government Maternity Hospital, Hyderabad in collaboration with Zudovidina from March 2000 to September 2001. The drug has to be given for a minimum period of four weeks. There were higher dropout cases and there were unregistered cases appeared after a period of 37 weeks to whom the drug was not given. Because the Government changed the drug to Nevirapine – a single dose therapy. This drug is supposed to very effective universally. But, however, the project officials agree that it is not possible to stop the transmission of the HIV virus from mother-to-child in every case as some children get infected with the virus in spite of the administration of Nevirapine.

An investigation has been conducted at the Hyderabad centre with regard to the effect of the drug. It is found that out of 118 Mother-Baby pairs received this drug under supervision four babies contacted the HIV virus. The *polymerised Chain Reaction Test* was conducted. This has correctly provided the result.

This test was conducted at the MGR University, Chennai. The Hyderabad centre had collected only the blood sample from the cases and sent to them. Medical scientists working on this problem are of the view that breast feeding was another important factor in the transmission of the AIDS. In spite of the administration of the drug Noverapine if the mother is an infected person and resort to breast feeding there might be transmission of the HIV virus to the child. Therefore, the infected mother should be prevented from breast feeding.

In one of the investigations it was found that about ten per cent of the pregnant women were found to be HIV positive at the Government Hospital of Vijayawada in a four months period. The officials stated that it is eight to ten per cent. But it is an alarming figure compared to any standard. The national average is two per cent, but the unofficial average is about 12 to 15 per cent. Vijayawada was having the largest number of HIV positive cases next to Mumbai in the country. The Aids Control Society has started a voluntary counselling and testing centre at Vijayawada. It is for all pregnant women going to the Government Hospitals for undergoing blood test after the counselling is made. Medicines are supplied to prevent the disease from being transmitted by the mother to her child (2002).

With all the efforts made by the AIDS Control Board and the Government of Andhra Pradesh to control the AIDS, people infected with the HIV positive were dying before proper medication reach them.

Here is case history reported by Melly Maitreyi (2002) from Hyderabad. The Andhra Pradesh High Court came for the rescue of a poor young women, Kamala, aged 28 years. She was a married woman, having a son aged 6 years. She was infected with HIV positive, lost her husband few years ago and also her son at the age of six few months ago. They died because of the dreaded disease, the Acquired Immune Deficiency Syndrome (AIDS).

Looking physically and mentally weak, Kamala had a smile on her face when The Hindu (Daily) Newspaper reporter met her two days after the Andhra Pradesh High Court had issued an order directing the State Government to provide her treatment and nourishment for fighting the AIDS. Kamala now had developed hopes and confidence to lead a normal life as long as possible, rather than to die as one among the millions deaths everyday. She has developed this hope in the midst of rude society, uncaring parents, siblings and in-laws. She was driven to the state of destitute and the court came for rescue at this stage. When she got married to a driver, she was healthy and happy. Her husband was a car driver first in 1995 and when he became a lorry driver, he was away from home for long time. His absence at home for long time was a secret, kept from Kamala and her family. After some time she developed health complaints and found her husband also fell sick often. A son was born at the time when she was in the spells of attacks in 1996.

She took her husband forcibly to the Osmania General Hospital and doctors after testing him declared that he is infected with HIV positive. Tests revealed that she and her son also were infected with the same virus. Kamala's in-laws had refused to accept the truth and instantly blamed her and not their son for the illness. The parents of her husband approached sorcerers to get rid of their son from the evil forces. Kamala observed that her husband's condition was becoming very serious when he has developed some skin infection and she forcibly took him to Gandhi Hospital, where he died in 1998. She has to meet the wrath of her in-laws for not carrying out their advice. They drove her from the house and she took refuge in her parents' home with her son.

It was a very difficult time for her since her in-laws did not help her. Her father, who has spent already to meet her medical expenses, had retired from his job and attended his own family. However, Kamala had determined to keep her son alive, took care of even some minor illness and took him to doctors. They were very much sympathetic for her pathetic condition. She cried with tears in her eyes "My son is the only reason for my existence and I had determined to save him".

Kamala approached the Andhra Mahila Sabha Legal Aid Centre and also the State Legal Services Authority to help her for getting her a share from the property of her in-laws for the treatment of her son. They refused to give her a share from the property.

She could not get the attention of her relatives and none came forward to help her. She had continued her fight with the help of the legal aid centre, but suffered a major blow by the death of her son. The High Court order came to her very late and she could not save her son. But she has determined to carry on with the treatment assured to her, now at the Freedom Foundation Society and with the help of the Andhra Pradesh State AIDS Control Society. She is thinking of adopting an orphan and make out a living by making use of her vocational skills even though her relatives literally waiting for her death.

HIV-AIDS IN TAMIL NADU - LATEST POSITION

Every State in India is organizing various programmes for fighting the epidemic and infectious diseases. The Government of Tamil Nadu had planned to launch a campaign for eradication of deliberating diseases which would reduce the productivity of the affected people. Though the life expectancy level in the State is increased, preventable diseases such as tuberculosis, pneumonia, cancer, malaria, leprosy, HIV/AIDS are persisting and serious consequences are caused. It is also distressing to know that malnutrition causes death of quite a number of children in the country, though sufficient amount of food is available. To end these pathetic conditions the State has launched an ambitious malnutrition-free Tamil Nadu programmes. These programmes started with multipurpose of eradicating the epidemic and infectious diseases and also diminishing the disease causing factors (2002). One of the important programmes is to fight the HIV/AIDS.

The preliminary part of the programme to fight the HIV-AIDS is making the people aware of the dreaded consequences. The AIDS awareness campaign is launched in various ways. The Voluntary Health Services (VHS) is launching specially designed van with messages to highlight the roll conditions in preventing infections. It is a touring van, will cover parts of Chennai City, Kanchipuram and Chengelpattu to create awareness about the spread of diseases like the HIV-AIDS (2002).

The Corporation Administration of Chennai has launched a campaign to create an awareness of the HIV-AIDS through autos. This programme was specially undertaken by the Chennai Corporation AIDS Prevention and Control Society. The 24 hours hot line counselling centre also was incorporated. It is widely held opinion that there are no correct and effective medicine to cure the HIV-AIDS disease. Therefore, one of the methods of attacking this dreaded disease is to create awareness about the prevention and management of the infection, which alone would be the solution to put an end to the menace. The hot line counselling centre has expressed that formerly cancer, tuberculosis and heart attacks were posing a major threat to the general public, but now it is the HIV-AIDS that endangers the lives of the people. It was also observed that the Medical Scientists must take it up as a challenge and face the deadliest disease and find out medicines and methods of treatment for eradicating the disease.

There are instances of death by hanging by the AIDS infected persons. The press reports run like this. One Manimaran aged forty was living in Kolathur a place close to Chennai. He had admitted himself in Tambaram Hospital for Tuberculosis treatment. Doctors examined him and found that he is HIV-AIDS infected person. Following this he was admitted in the AIDS wards and was taking the treatment. On knowing that he is suffering from the AIDS, Manimaran hanged himself in a tree in the Hospital complex and died. Police investigations were made and it was known that he was mentally broken for having infected with the AIDS and felt ashamed of it and decided to end his life. Following this incidence, another person, who was living in Tambaram area, named Balaji, aged twenty committed suicide and died in his house. On investigation, he was mentally upset on knowing that he had the HIV-AIDS disease. There were also unreported AIDS deaths by committing suicide, Mishimizu also examined many NGO and Government run AIDS interventions.

The recent information about the AIDS in Tamil Nadu is very much astounding. This is reported by Sujatha (2002) to the *Hindu* on November 30th, 2002, under the heading of 'State tops in AIDS cases'. According to this report Tamil Nadu tops the list of States in India with 18,276 cases reported till the August 2002, which is very much ahead of Maharashtra State, which accounts for 8,262 AIDS cases.

According to a report by the National AIDS Control Programme Tamil Nadu accounts for nearly 46 per cent of the total number of AIDS cases reported to the National AIDS Control Organization. In the State, the Capital city, Chennai is having the largest number of cases with 6,060 of which 4,591 are AIDS infected male patients. In the State, Nilgiris is having the lowest number of cases 39. Of the total number of cases reported, the addresses of 312 patients are not known.

The number of patients died of this disease is 185 in the year 2002 alone. The Deputy Director of Tamil Nadu State AIDS Control Society has reported that there are about 500 patients in the risk age group of 20-39 years. They are found to be infected with the HIV positive. These persons constitute 96 per cent of the total number of cases. These persons were involved in indiscriminate sexual (promiscuity) activities. Out of the total number of cases the prenatal transmission cases of the HIV virus are accounted for 3.15 per cent. The admission cases are consistently increasing in the Hospitals.

CHILDREN PRE-DATED IN THE FLESH TRADE IN INDIA

The emergence of the AIDS in India and its consequences has brought to light several sex related problems. Apart from the adult women and adolescent girls involved in sex trade, the innocent children also are found to be involved in flesh trade. It is estimated that about six lakhs of children in India are being predated in the flesh trade. Children constitute fifteen per cent of the prostitutes in India. The children involved in sex trade are from six major cities of Delhi, Mumbai, Kolkata, Hyderabad, Bangalore and Chennai, the total comes to one lakh. This makes an average of sixteen thousand children in Chennai. This being the case, either the Government of Tamil Nadu or the Chennai police are not having any record of the incidence of this children sex trade (*City Mag*, Vol-40, July 7, 2002).

The Chennai city police make many raids and arrests quite a large number of young women and girls in their late teen ages. The *City Mag* states that when questioned, there was only callous attitude and indifferent answers obtained from them. It was a shocking information reported in some dailies that Policemen run sex trade and they were arrested. (*Thanti*, October, 2002). The Government of Tamil Nadu issued a notification requesting the contestants of the local body elections to address the problem of child prostitution on assuming power. It is also brought to the attention of the public that the Government is appointing "watch dog" committees in collaboration with the local representatives in selected cities all over Tamil Nadu to prevent the child sex trade.

There were also seminars on Inter-State Cross Trafficking of children. There are committees, met in Chennai, Madurai, Salem and Tiruchirapalli to check the child prostitution. With all these efforts child sex trade is still continuing in Chennai. It is the opinion of some people that the practice of child abuse goes back to the period of *Devadasi* culture which was called the "*debauched primitiveness of India*", by the British Parliament in 1885. The National Commission for Women in Tamil Nadu had conducted a survey and revealed that many of them were survivors of incest. These people entered in sex trade out of shame, denial and hostility of the society and needs for survival. But most of the children according to the said theory, follow their mothers, already in the sex trade. It is very pathetic and cruel that social tradition prevents the children of prostitutes from the public schools. As a result of it they are unskilled and unqualified for other jobs and therefore, there is no other go except to take up the sex trades at the earliest age. In this way, determined by the social customs and tradition the girl child takes up the mother's job and the boy becomes pimp for his mother and sister. There begins the risk of the epidemic and HIV-AIDS infections.

With regard to HIV-AIDS, Tamil Nadu is the State where the HIV-AIDS is reported as the first and has the highest level of HIV positive infected cases. The law drives the victims to a greater distance. The Prevention of Immoral Traffic Act (PITA) in force at present lays down that prostituting oneself is not punishable act, but soliciting in public is a punishable act or behaviour. This act is highly ambiguous. As a result of this any woman may be arrested on a charge of solicitation and punished. Astrayed Law executors may arrest any innocent girl or woman and can be penalized.

It is estimated that there are about six thousand to seven thousand children in India, might have experienced sexual abuse, mostly by the members of their own families. But it is very unfortunate that only one in hundred child abuse is reported. A report from Mumbai is that a majority of adolescent abortion seekers in Mumbai are the victims of rape and incest. The number of cases may be alarming if we go deep into this problem. These cases are increasing everywhere because of the premarital permissive promiscuous sexual activities. The motion picture themes which are highly obscene, easily tempt and insticate the adolescent boys and girls for illicit sex relations. These boys and girls once they taste the pleasures of sex they go rampantly and indiscriminately with the sexual activities. This may lead to seeking multiple partners in sexual activities. As a result of it infection of sexually transmitted diseases are not ruled out.

Urgent Need : The Fight of HIV-AIDS in India

It is felt that the grassroots projects are the key to deal with the AIDS successfully. The National AIDS Control Organization (NACO) has estimated that there are four million HIV infected persons in India. The main concentration of infection in India is on those who are poor and the marginal groups. There is great concern that the rate of HIV infection is about one per cent in spite of intervention programmes. This may increase to five per cent (37 millions) among the adults population. Stating the magnitude of the problem, Edwin Lim (2002), the World Bank's Country Director, states that fighting the HIV-AIDS in India requires urgent and continuous efforts. He further states that it also requires strengthened partnerships between the Government, the private sector, non-Governmental Organizations, donors and the international health community.

The fifth National Highway is running through the Southern

Indian State of Tamil Nadu. There is a halting point at Red Hills which caters to about six hundred truck drivers every day, who used to pull trucks off the road for rest and for eating a meal. It also serves as a classroom in which Santhoshi Social Service Research and Welfare Society, teaches, truck drivers, mechanical and local sex workers about the HIV-AIDS and other sexually transmitted diseases (STDs) and provides STD counselling and referrals. The NGO trusts on poor educators, namely former truck drivers and sex workers to motivate these high risk groups to change their behaviour and practice safe sex activities.

The World Bank's HIV-AIDS Control Project-II, represents the second commitment by the Bank to HIV-AIDS work being undertaken by India and brought the Bank's total support to 275 million Dollars. The Bank's South Asia Region also supports investments in HIV prevention and control in Bangladesh, Pakistan and Sri Lanka in HIV prevention (AAN-2002).

The major component of the project should be focussed on the high-risk groups – the commercial sex workers, truck drivers, migrant labourers, homosexual men and injecting drug users by providing poor counselling, condom promotion and treatment of STDs. The project also covers preventive interventions that will benefit the general community, including information and awareness campaigns, voluntary testing and counselling and STD clinics, and efforts to reduce transmission through blood transfusions and occupational exposure.

Further, for providing the low-cost treatment for the people of the AIDS infected, the project provides funds home-based and community-based care, including increased access to cost-effective interventions for common opportunistic infections such as tuberculosis, pneumonia and cancer. On the basis of the earlier effort the project will help to strengthen the effectiveness and technical, managerial and financial sustainability of national, state and municipal programmes. This is to expand and improve nationwide STD-HIV-AIDS surveillance and for data collection and to increase national research capacity.

While addressing the Fifth International Conference on AIDS in Asia in Kuala Lumpur, Mieka Nishimiz has stated that AIDS threatened South Asia, not in generations, not in decades, not in years, but now today. It is not an exaggeration, but AIDS threatens the security and stability of the nation. It is not like any other disease and not just a public health matter, but it is a singularly most critical, socio-economic development issue in India, for which financial assistance is provided from the World Bank, to the campaign like the one "Red Hills" to know more about India's efforts to fight the AIDS.

The AIDS Counselling Centre in New Delhi is located in Safdarjung Hospital. It is a Government Hospital and people from lower income groups mostly go to this Hospital and receive counselling on AIDS. At the Tambaram Tuberculosis Institute for Thoracic Medicine in Chennai about forty per cent of all the patients admitted are HIV positive and there are 540 patients of AIDS infected in the hospital, in the advanced stage of this disease. The patients admitted here represent a spectrum of people infected by HIV-AIDS from housewives and children to truck drivers and transvestites. The patients were talking about AIDS awareness and told that they carry the messages and spread out them when they get rid of the disease and return to their homes.

According to Nishimizu the most important component of the effective design of preventive programme is listening to the perspective of those who are infected with the HIV positive. It was also observed that at the Community Health Education Society (CHES) the commercial sex workers are now actively involved in educating their co-workers/peers on how to prevent HIV-AIDS, introspecting into their past experiences. The society provides also homes for children, who are infected with AIDS and to those who have been abandoned by their parents-families. In the red-light area Sonagachi, District of Calcutta, sex workers with the support of the Government and NGOs have organized themselves and created a task force to promote the use of condoms in commercial sex activities. It is known that the use of condom raised from three per cent in 1992 to over ninety per cent in 1998. Another improved preventive information is that in Mumbai the HIV infection was fifty per cent among the commercial sex workers previously and the same was brought down to five per cent (AAN, 2002).

own financial cooperatives. They started becoming literates, have organized to demanding protection from the Police abuses and also are preventing forced child prostitution. There is a start for sustained social transmission, which may promote the human dignity and the quality of life.

Bibliography

Action Plan on AIDS, *The Hindu*, September 8, 2002.

AIDS, Threatening India, *Daily Thanthi*, October 3, 2002.

AIDS Awareness, *The Hindu*, September 9, 16, 2002.

Akars, R. : Teenage drinking and drug use. In E.D. Evans, Ed., *Adolescents : Readings in Behaviour Development,* Hindale, III; Dryten, 1970.

Asha Nehemiah : Fighting AIDS with awareness, Sunday Magazine, *Indian Express,* September 8, 1991.

Banerjea, D., Latest Findings on AIDS and its Treatment, *Everyman's Science*, XXVII (1), February-March, 1992, pp. 7-12.

Baron, R.A., and Byrne, D., *Social and Psychology* (5th Ed.,) New Delhi, Prentice-Hall of India Private Limited, 1988.

Bartell, G.D., Group Sex Among the Mid-Americans, *Journal of Sex Research*, 1970, 6, 113-130.

Bennett, W. The Nicotine fix, *Harvard Magazine,* 1980, 82, 10-14.

Bhattacharya, A., Manipur in the Tightening Grip of 'AIDS', *Probe India,* October, 1990, 71-73.

Boehm, G., At last a nonaddicting substitute for morphine? *Today's Health*, 1968, 46, (4), 69-72.

Byrne, D., Lamberth, J. : The effect of erotic stimuli on sex arousal, evaluative responses and subsequent behaviour. In technical report of the Commission on Obscenity and Pornography, Vol. 8, Washington D.C. US. Government Printing Press, 1971.

Carsaon, R.C., Butcher, J.N., Coleman, J.C., *Abnormal Psychology and Modern Life*. Scott, Forceman and Co., London, 1988.

City Mag. Children Predated in the flesh trade in India. Vol. 40 July 26. 2002.

Clement, U. Schmidt, G., and Kruse, M. : Changes in Sex differences in sexual behaviour : A replication of a study on West German Students (1966-1981). *Archives of Sexual Behaviour,* 1984, 13, 99-120.

Coleman, J.C., and Broen., W.B.: *Abnormal Psychology and Modern Life,* Bombay : D.B. Taraporevala Sons & Co., Private Limited., 1972.

Chennai, HIV Counsellors Have Few Ready Answers. *The Times of India.*, 1995, July.

Collins English Dictionary, London : Collins, 1979.

Cooper, R., *Sleep*, New York : Champman and Hall Medical, 1994.

Davison, G.C., and Neale, J.M. : *Abnormal Psychology* (5th Ed.,) New York : John Wiley & Sons, 1990.

Express News Service, 27 HIV Positive in 20 days, *Indian Express*, October 13, 1991.

Fawcet, J. Y. : *Psychology and Population,* New York : The Population Council, 245, Park Avenue, 1970.

Fort J.P. : Jr. Heroin addict among young men. *Psychiatry,* 1954, 17, 251-259.

Ford, A.B., Casualties of our time. *Science*, 1970, 167, 156-263.

Gabel, R.H., Barnard, N., Norke, M., and O'Connell, R.A., AIDS Presenting as Mania, *Comprehensive Psychiatry*, 1986, 27, 251-54.

Gates, United States AIDS Programme, Medical Science. *The Hindu*, October 6, 2001.

Gilmartin, B.G., That Swinging Couple Down the Block, *Psychology Today,* 1975, 8 (9) 54.

Glenn, N.D., and Weaver, C.N. : Attitudes toward premarital, extramarital and homosexual relations in the U.S. in the 1970s. *Journal of Sex Research*, 1979, 15, 108-118.

Goode, E., *The Marijuana Smokers.* New York : Basic Books, 1970. Government Hospital, Chennai.

Greer, S. Cancer and the Mind, *British Journal of Psychiatry* 1993, 143, 535-543.

H.O.D., Rota, T., Schooley, R., Kaplan. J., Allen. J., Groopman, J., Resnick. L., Felsenstein, L., Andrews, C., and Hirsch, M. : Isolation of HTLV-III from cerebrospinal fluid and neural tissues of patients with neurologic symptoms related to the acquired immune deficiency syndrome (AIDS). *New England Journal of Medicine*, 1985, 313, 1493-1497.

Hunt, M., *Sexual Behaviour in the 1970s*. Chicago : Playboy Press, 1974.

Innocents Interrupted, *City Mag.*, Vol. 40, July 26, 2002.

Ibrahim, A. The Home Situation and the Homosexual, *Journal of Sex Research*, 1976, 12, 263-282.

Jacob John. : No part of India free of infection (an interview by Asha) Sunday Magazine, *Indian Express,* September 8, 1991.

Jaffe, H., Drug addiction and drug abouse, In Goodman and Gilman's *The Pharmacological Basis of Therapeutic Behaviour*, New York : Macmillan, Co., 1985.

Jemmott, J.B., & Lock, S.E., Psychosocial factors, Immunologic medication and Human Susceptibility to infectious disease. How much do we know? *Psychological Bulletin*, 1984, 95, 79-108.

Keeler, M.H. : Motivation and marijuana use : a correlate of adverse reaction, *American Journal of Psychiatry*, 1968, 125, 386-390.

Kelley, K., *Females, Males and Sexuality*, Albany, New York; State University of New York Press, 1986.

Klein, D.N., Depue, R.A., & Slater, J.F. Inventory identification of Cyclothemia : IX. Validation in Offspring of Bipolar patient. *Arch., Gen., Psychiatry,* 1986, 43, 441-45.

Kemble, J., *Idols and Invalids*, New York : Doubleday, 1936.

Kolb, B., and Wishaw, Jan Q., *Fundamentals of Human Neuropsychology*, (4th Ed.,) New York : N.W.A. Freeman and Company, 1996.

Kowlas, L., 2000, Creation of an HIV/AIDS Database : Perspectives and Possibilities, International Conference on Science, Technology and Mathematics Education for Human Development, Goa, India : CASTME-UNESCO-HBCSE, February 20-23, 2001, p. 173.

Letters : Depth of Degeneration, *Indian Express,* Madras, October 24th, 1991.

Liebert, R.M., Poulos, R.M. and Strauss, C.D. : *Developmental Psychology*, Englewood Cliffs, New Jersey : Prentice-Hall, INC., 1974.

Mani, R.S., A Study of Health Awareness of Secondary and Higher Secondary Teacher Trainees and Higher Secondary Students, U.G.C. Minor Research Project, Vadodara : CASE, The M.S. University of Baroda, 2001.

Marathe, K., Let It Be We Will Both Die Together, *The Times of India*, 1995, August 6.

McCandless,, B.R. : *Adolescents, Behaviour and Development, Hinsdale,* HI: Dryton, 1970.

Medical Science, can HIV be filtered from patients' blood? *The Hindu,* July 12, 2001.

Medical Science, *The Hindu*, September 2, 2002.

Medical Science, *The Hindu*, September 5, 2002.

Medical Science, *The Hindu*, August 3, 2002.

Melly, Meitrayi, M.C. Court Comes to her rescue, Chennai : *The Hindu*, September 7, 2002.

Michale, Merson : AIDS and the Status of Women, *Tehran Times International Weekly*, December 13, 1990.

Navia, B.A., Cho, E., Petito, C.K., and Price, R.W. : The AIDS dementia complex : II : Neuropathology, *Annals of Neurology*, 1986, 19, 525-535.

New Scientist, *The Hindu.*

Nietzal, M.T., *et al.*, : Behavioural Approach to Community Psychology, New York : Pergaman Press, 1977.

Nurnberg, H.G., Prudic., J., Fiori, M., and Freeman, E. : Psychopathology Complicating Acquired Immune Deficiency Syndrome (AIDS) *American Journal of Psychiatry,* 1984, 141, 95-96.

Pal, S. Fifty four per cent of Drug Addicts might turn out to be AIDS positive, *Probe India,* October, 1990, 74-77.

Parran, T., Shadow on the land, New York : Reynal and Hitchcock Hitchcock, 1937.

Philiprice, F., *Marriage and Parenthood,* Allyn and Bacon Inc. Boston, 1979.

Phillips, D.E. and Gromko, M.H. : Sex differences in sexual activity : Reality or illusion? *Journal of Sex Research* 1985, 21, 437-448.

Pusey, W.A., *The History of Epidemiology of Syphilis*, Springfield : Charles C. Thomas, 1933.

Pushpa Khurana, AIDS : *Humanities Gravest Challenge*, New Delhi : Hind Pocket Books, 1989.

Rajamanickam, M. Psycho-Social Study of the AIDS and the drug abuses, *Journal of Community Guidance and Research*, 1992, 9(1), January, pp. 17-42.

Ronald De Pinho, Cancer Development in Older Adults, Medical Science, *The Hindu,* January 11, 2001.

Sadhukhan, R.K., A.K. Halder and S.L. Chakraborty, Some Immunological Aspects of AIDS, *Everyman's Science*, 1992-93, XXVII(6), December - January, pp. 193-195.

Snadhya Nammalwar : AIDS threat looms large over Tamil Nadu' *Indian Express*, October 13, 1991.

Science Express Service, Child AIDS cases soring, *Indian Express,* February 10, 1991.

Science Notes, DDI : A second AIDS drug, *Indian Express,* October 27, 1991.

Sibnath Deb., Rehabilitation of the Children of Commercial Sex Workers Through Participatory Approach, *Journal of Community Guidance and Research*, 2002, 193, 299-314.

Siegelman, M. Parental Background of Male Homosexuals and Heterosexuals, *Archives of Sexual Behaviours*, 1974, 3, 3-18.

Snider, V.D., Simpson, D.M., Nielson, E., Gold, J.W.M., Metroka, C.K., and Posner, J.B., Neurological complications of acquired immune deficiency syndrome : Analysis of 50 patients, *Annals of Neurology*, 1983, 14, 403-468.

Srinivasan, V. *Health Update Multiple Perspectives on Health Empowerment,* 3 (12), August, 1999.

Stott, H.L. : *The Psychology of Human Development*, Delhi : The Macmillan Company of India Limited, 1974.

Strange, J.R., *Abnormal Psychology*, Bombay : TATA McGraw Hill Publishing Company Ltd., 1965.

Suresh, N. : Checking AIDS – The Indian Way. *The Times of India*, February, 1991.

Sujatha, R. State Tops in AIDS Cases, *The Hindu,* November 30, 2002.

Telegraph Group Limited, London; *The Hindu*, 2002.

Ultmann, M., Belman, A., Ruff, H., Novick, B., Cone-Weason, B., Cohen, H., and Rubinstein, A. : Development abnormalities in children with Acquired Immune Deficiency Syndrome (AIDS) and AIDS-related complex. *Developmental Medicine and Child Neurology* 1985, 27, 563-571.

Urgent Need to fight AIDS in India, Ambattur-Annanagar, *Weekend,* August, 31, 2002.

Venkoba B. Rao, A., : AIDS and Health Education Sciences Express, *Indian Express,* November 30, 1990.

Vicent, R.J. : Investigation of attitudes of eighth, tenth and twelfth grade students towards smoking marijuana, Dissertation Abstracts, 1989, 29, 3799-3800.

Walk, D.K. Youth and Drugs. : Guidelines for teachers, *Social Education,* 1969, 44, 667-674.

Werner, K.L. The effects of the antismoking campaign on cigarette consumption, *American Journal of Public Health*, 1977, 6, 645-650.

INDEX